# The MammySlammy

# The MammySlammy

✦

## Mammograms with Courage and Humor

*Sharon Marler*

iUniverse, Inc.
New York  Lincoln  Shanghai

# The MammySlammy
## Mammograms with Courage and Humor

iUniverse, Inc.


For information address:
iUniverse, Inc.
2021 Pine Lake Road, Suite 100
Lincoln, NE 68512
www.iuniverse.com


ISBN: 0-595-27074-3

Printed in the United States of America

# Contents

# *Acknowledgements*

Love and appreciation to
Dick, my dearest friend, who became my love,
And to Leisl and Melissa, our daughters,
Who gave our lives meaning as they taught us what is important and
what is not.


The Butties—Chris, Julie, Kay, and Vicki
for giving new definition to friendship, and to
Eliz and John…for encouraging personal growth.

To those Great Friends who make work
a fun game to play…
too many to list them all.


To the many people in my life who
have helped me learn to reach out,
and more importantly, to recognize
the helping hands that reach in.


To those who fought cancer and won.
In Memory of those who lost their battle
And to their loved ones left behind.

And,
To my elusive Comforter-Friend,
real or imagined,
who still guides my life.

# *Introduction*

Fear and denial. Two strong emotions that can mean life or death to anyone who ignores preventative health care. The mammogram is a much-feared and often-denied diagnostic tool that can detect early signs of breast cancer and save the lives of thousands of women every year. Worries that it is uncomfortable—if not downright painful—not to mention embarrassing, makes it an easy test for many women to avoid—until it is too late.

Sharon Marler knows the hurdles that all women must leap on their way to having a mammogram. Even after having survived breast cancer, she once struggled with making an appointment to have this all-important test done.

Fortunately, Sharon has two rare gifts—a fabulous sense of humor and a creative mind. She exemplifies "thinking outside of the box." Instead of living in dread of having a mammogram done, she found a way to make it fun for herself and her friends. She invented the MammySlammy.

The MammySlammy is the subject of this book. It is Sharon's way of turning her profound and life-changing battle with breast cancer into a catalyst to help other women and their families stop cancer in its tracks, or, to handle it if it has advanced to a late stage.

MammySlammy is about love. Love of oneself, one's family, and of life at its deepest, darkest days and its lightest, most joyful moments. Read it with an open mind, design your own MammySlammy, and make taking charge of your health an exciting adventure for yourself and your friends.

Elizabeth Laden, Author of Angels of the Unborn,
and Mystic Warriors of the Yellowstone
Island Park, ID.
February 2003

# Saying NO to Breast Cancer

One by one, cars pulled into the parking lot. Doors opened, and women stepped out of their cars, tentatively, expectantly. Some were as anxious as they were on their wedding night or when they gave birth to their first child. Some were so afraid they could barely speak. All had dug deep inside themselves to that place where their life experiences had taught them to store up extra courage and spiritual strength. It was time for their mammograms!

Some hesitated, wondering if all the horror stories were true. You know the stories: *Open the fridge door, place your breast against the door-frame, and have a two-thousand pound giant slam the door on you and then lean against it. Lie down on the cold floor of the garage, place your breast under the back tire, and have some one drive your car across it.* And, so on, and so on. Funny little jokes we use to put ourselves at ease; unrealistic concepts that make us laugh uncomfortably and add another dose of fear to getting a Mammogram.

Each one looked around, taking in her surroundings, as she questioned her instinct to get back in her car and flee. Bravely, each decided to go ahead with it, but the questions remained.

*Will it hurt?*
*Isn't it embarrassing?*
*How private is it?*
*Will I feel violated?*
*Who actually handles my breast?*
*Will it make me feel, you know? Creepy?*

The questions go on and on.

Each woman reached back into her car for her purse, a necessary item, and for the gift she had brought to this strange party, wondering if it was an appropriate gift for the occasion. And, wondering if partici-pating in this occasion was appropriate at all. *A MammySlammy Party. I must be crazy to even be here.*

Each walked to the door of the Imaging Center, and entered with relief that she wasn't the first one to arrive. Sharon was there, and so were others. Whew! That was a relief! No one likes to be alone.

The waiting room of the Imaging Center was comfortably decorated in early 'let's make our clients as comfortable as they can be under the circumstances' décor. The gentle color scheme invoked relaxation. Each woman checked in with the receptionist who verified her infor-mation, matching names to doctor scripts and insurances. Then, each was invited back to the party room for the day's activities.

The party room was decorated with helium-filled bright pink bal-loons. Gifts began to adorn the built-in side board against the south wall of the room. A large table surrounded by chairs sat in the middle of the room for those important family/client and doctor conferences. The table sported a cake, plates, utensils, snacks, and party sacks. A multi-media cart supported a TV and a VCR in the corner of the room. A door opened from the party room to a hallway where the rest rooms, dressing rooms, and examining rooms were located.

Each woman would be called on to go through the door, down the hallway, into the dressing room and then to the examining room on her own. Each would open her own door to ensuring she would increase her chances of never having a cancer story to tell.

# *Opening the Door*

## A MammySlammy Party Day

Understand right from the beginning that having a MammySlammy Party does not, and will not, diminish the importance of yearly mammograms. It is not intended to make it a joke, embarrass anyone, nor give avenue for making it a crude, uncaring time.

A MammySlammy is a planned event to ensure health, give support, and build friendships. It is held to lessen the anxiety of those who fear or procrastinate having a mammogram. Treat the occasion respectfully and joyfully.

## What? Who? Where? When? Why? How?

It is easy to explain the 'what'. The 'why' is full of complex emotions, each experienced by individuals, but in many different ways.

## What:

A MammySlammy is a shared occurrence of making the necessary, worrisome, and occasionally uncomfortable experience of having a mammogram a more pleasant event. Together, women visit, play games, perhaps watch a "chick-flick", exchange gifts, share information and stories, solve all the problems of the world, and solidify the bond of friendship as they fight the war against breast cancer.

Other than cancers of the skin, breast cancer is the most common cancer for women. In 2001, over 192,000 cases of invasive breast cancer were diagnosed.

Another 47,000 women were diagnosed with *in situ,* or confined, cancers that have not spread beyond the area where they began. Most cases of in situ cancers are detectable only through mammography.

Although there has been a decline in breast cancer mortality, breast cancer claimed the lives of over 40,000 women in 2001. The decline in mortality has been attributed to the improvements in breast cancer treatments over the past years and to the availability of mammography screening.

Early detection, when breast cancers are either *in situ* or in early stages of invasive disease, is essential in fighting this disease. Remember, mammography screening can identify cancer several years before physical symptoms develop.

## Who:

MammySlammy is a gathering of women

- who love life,
- who care for one another's well-being,
- who want to ensure their good health
- who want to ensure a quality life
- who know how to make the best of life
- who will be there to cheer when the mammogram shows no evidence of breast cancer, or
- who will be a strong support group should cancer be detected.

## Where:

Most hospitals or imaging centers have a training room or education room that can be used. Call around to see who will work with you.

## When:

Annually. October is national Breast Cancer Awareness month, but any time that works best in your location is a great time to hold a MammySlammy.

Our group has been holding ours in June. The 2002 MammySlammy was held in concert with the Relay for Life Walkathon, and with the last month of the fiscal year most of us deal with before needing to meet our insurance company deductible—again.

I think we will gradually move ours to October to give more focus to the entire breast cancer awareness in our area.

## Why:

The *why* is more difficult for me to explain. Perhaps an explanation of why I hosted the first MammySlammy will help to define the "why".

I am a breast cancer survivor who strongly believes in regular medical check-ups, including the annual mammogram. I knew I was due for a mammogram. No, that isn't quite true. I realized that I had become comfortable with being a survivor and didn't want to risk becoming a victim once again. I just didn't want to think about cancer, so I had foolishly avoided getting a mammogram for two-plus years. I knew it wasn't smart to be avoiding such a simple, life-saving thing; yet, I couldn't make myself pick up the phone and call to make an appointment.

I justified this foolishness by reasoning that I was healthy, had no signs of a problem, and I was too busy to get it done right then. It was easy to put it off until later. Besides, I never said I *wasn't* going to do it. I planned to make an appointment sometime…later…when I could.

Honesty always has a way of reaching through the surface front. Truth soon forced me to admit that I was afraid to face the possibility that there could be a return of cancer. After all, when I was in the hospital after surgery, I promised God that I would not ask for anything more if only my life would be extended so I could see my children raised to be adults. Here I was with an empty nest and the haunting thought that payment could be due soon. I was just too scared to do it alone.

Fortunately, I had a group of friends—Julie, Vicki, Kay, and Chris—to turn to. We had been drawn together through involvement in a professional association and have remained friends throughout the years. I called Julie and asked her if she had been in for her yearly mammogram. She said she had not. I suggested we go together and make it a party. We laughed, then contacted Kay, Vicki, and Chris—our cohorts in adventure—and invited them to our party. All, of course, agreed that:

1) it was a sensible thing to do, and

2) it was as good a reason for a party as anything else we could think of at the time.

I called the Imaging Center in Idaho Falls and asked if they had a party room we could use. Kathy, who answered the phone, hesitated a moment, then said, "Do you have the right number?"

"Is this the Imaging Center?"

"Yes, it is," she answered.

"Then, I have the right place."

I knew I had to 'sell' the idea of making mammograms a party! I explained that a group of us wanted to come in together and make getting a mammogram a joyful, rather than anxious, occasion. We wanted to make it a party, a celebration of sorts. We would need a room big enough to hold all of us along with cake, goodies, balloons, and gifts. We would be playing games and may get a little loud, so it would be wonderful if we had a room that was isolated from the rest of their clients.

Kathy got Wendy to join us on the phone line, and I was asked to, once again, explain what our group wanted to do. They said they loved the idea of making it a party and we were off to planning out the details of the event. They agreed to allow us to use the education room at the center, and said we could invite even more than the five of us if we would like to do so. That sounded good to me.

I told Kathy and Wendy that those we invited would identify themselves as the *MammySlammy Group*. The Imaging Center's staff were absolutely great to work with. Together we selected a date, reserved timeslots and the party was on the way to realization.

I also invited the wonderful group of friends that I work with to attend the party—Kate, Sara, Bobbe, Bonnie, Kelly, and Kathy. This was going to be a fun thing to do together.

## How:

Now I was faced with not knowing what others would expect from a MammySlammy Party. Would frivolity lessen the importance of what we were doing, or would it take the sting out of the worry and anxiety? What could be done to keep everyone involved while one or two at a time rotated from involvement in a game or activity to the examining room and back in to the game or activity again? How could we make everyone blend so no one felt left out, anxious or uncomfortable? It was easy to do with the five of us...we knew each other well and loved spending time together.

What if one invited someone that another didn't like? That could create an unpleasant stress. It was all getting too complicated until I realized that we were all adults and if we didn't know how to play fair with one another, it was time to learn to do so. Who knows, the MammySlammy could even become the common ground on which anger problems and misunderstandings between women could find a medium of tolerance, care and concern and, hopefully, a resolve of forgiveness and new friendship.

The first year MammySlammy was an uncertain adventure, to say the least, but I knew it would be a way to ensure annual mammograms. And I knew this would be a way to make it fun—parties are made to be fun! Friends, love, and laughter are what add value to our lives. She who laughs—lasts.

The first thing I would recommend is to know what is going on in your community at the time. Is there a new restaurant where you could eat? Is there a movie, definitely chick flick quality, or a theatre presentation that you could attend together after the MammySlammy party? Is there a live concert that you could all get tickets to? Is there a walk-a-thon in which you could all participate? Find out what is going on in the area and use anything that is pleasant to attach to the Mammy-Slammy party. It is rather like the song in Mary Poppins: "a spoon full of sugar makes the medicine go down." Hold a 1950s theme party and Rock and Roll those blues away. Take the ideas given, modify them to meet your needs, or use your own new and innovative ideas to make your parties memorable. Take photographs of the attendees and build a Sisterhood of the MammySlammy scrapbook that can be updated yearly. Realize that the party needs to fit you, your friends both old and new, and the resources that are available for you to use.

## The Basics:

Get yourself in a party mood. Realize that you are the catalyst for changing how the annual mammogram is anticipated. Be excited! Step forward and take the lead. You can be a positive instrument of change.

More importantly, you can provide a vital step in early detection of breast cancer. You are not only stepping forward to protect yourself, but you are ensuring your friends are around to enjoy life with you. Make attendance at the MammySlammy a fun and a fashionable thing to do.

Call the imaging center, clinic or hospital where you are going to schedule your appointments, tell them what you want to do, and ask if they would be willing to let you use a private waiting area/room where you and your friends can have a get-together. (Take them a copy of the MammySlammy book.)

You have the room. You have the date. What next?

- Contact your closest friends.
- Tell them you value their positive influence on your life.
- Ask them if they have had their annual mammogram.
- Tell them you have scheduled a *celebration of life party* called a MammySlammy, and would like them to join you on (date and time).
- Ask if they will make their annual appointment for the designated day.
- Help them get enthusiastically involved in the planning and sharing.
- Ask for their ideas on what to do. Seek out new and fresh ideas for your party.
- Most importantly, once they commit to being involved, encourage them to invite others.
- Suggest you go to breakfast or lunch together before your appointments.
- Set the mood for fun, support, and camaraderie.
- Have each attendee bring a gift that pertains to the event.
- Let attendees select and open a gift when they have completed their mammogram.
- Then have the person who brought the gift tell why they selected that particular gift.

We have had gag gifts that made us all laugh and realize that life is fun. We have had gifts from the heart that remind us that life is dear and friendships are treasured. There have been sharing of recipes, favorite books or movies, beautiful throws or pillows for comfort, colognes and bubble bath for relaxations, and many other wonderful items. The list is as extensive as all things imagined. Whatever you choose to do, make sure your MammySlammy is a *celebration of life*, memorable for all.

Above all, <u>do</u> <u>not</u> set a price range for the gift purchase. This is not about dollars-and-cents; it is about feelings, sharing, and enjoying one another's company. There is no price tag on friendship. It isn't a 'fair exchange' of dollar value. It is about gifts from the heart, from the soul, given without monetary measurement attached.

Another suggestion is to work collectively to make something special for someone not there. Like what?

Well, you could set up quilting frames and tie a quilt for someone currently on chemo therapy. Have everyone bring a toy and an article of clothing for a child and put together Christmas Boxes. Bring new warm nightgowns, fleece throws, or slippers to donate to a nursing home. Bring care packages filled with items needed for a safe house or shelter for women(check with them and see what is needed). Consider bringing food baskets to give to shelters, needy, etc.

Wow! So many things are possible when a caring group meets together. Being actively involved in doing something for someone else builds inner strength and increases personal self worth. Dare to share.

Whatever you choose to do, make sure you plan a closing ceremony that gives participants renewed courage, knowledge of self and others, and awareness of the role they play in bringing joy and happiness to their inner beings as well as to the lives of others.

Last year I took in early invitation cards for next year's Mammy-Slammy. I presented each attendee with an invitation and a candle-holder that held three small candles. I asked them to arrange some time for solitude and reflection where they could light a candle for someone who was a cancer survivor, one for someone who did not survive cancer, and one for themselves for having the courage to preserve their health and peace of mind.

I asked them to resolve to bring two friends to the next Mammy-Slammy Party, and to write the names of these friends on the invitation as a promise that they would share the idea with others.

Ideas for a MammySlammy party are as numerous as the number of women who need mammograms. There are games to invent and play, movies to watch, books to discuss, and stories to write. Hold a *Show-and-Tell MammySlammy*. Show, discuss, and share something you do well; i.e., did you write a poem? Did you run a race? Play with a child? Go for a long leisure walk? Take a photograph? Whatever you did, acknowledge the worth of it. Plan a *Share-and-Glow MammySlammy* where each attendee is asked to bring health tips, favorite poems and books, best jokes, and whatever else would fit into the category of the day.

How about A Year in the Life of a Slammer theme? Give all attendees a MammySlammy journal and ask them to write their everyday thoughts, challenges, opportunities and achievements for the coming year, and bring it to share at the next party. Above all, remember to make the "Hurrahs" loud and appreciative.

Make your MammySlammy be an annual retreat from a hectic world. Make it a 'girl talk' time of sharing, planning, laughing and just being together. Plan it out, but don't be too surprised if the day takes to its own road. They have a tendency to do that. Just rely on instinct and follow where it takes you.

Be sure to keep a record of what worked at the party, and what did not. Collect ideas from others, and most of all, share your ideas with others. I'd love to hear your suggestions and successes. Please take a minute to share them with me: Sharon Marler, P O Box 105, St. Anthony ID 83445 or by email at **smarler@srv.net**. Ideas and stories will be posted on the MammySlammy website—**www.mammyslammy.com**

Let me share with you now what we East Idahoans have done at our MammySlammy parties.

# *The Party*

## Year 1: Our new adventure

We didn't know what to do for our first party. In fact, we didn't know that this would be so much fun and such an easy way to do the annual glamour shot, that it would become a yearly event.

We did know we had a marvelous new Italian restaurant in Idaho Falls so that is where we met for lunch. We gathered at the restaurant at 11:30 a.m. and spent over an hour getting acquainted, sharing girl talk, and eating absolutely delicious main course garlic foods, followed with that melt in your mouth tira misu dessert.

"This is a great idea…I think."

"Can you believe we let Sharon talk us into this?"

"Do we open gifts here or what?"

"No, let's wait until we are all through getting slammed."

"What do we do next?"

"This is my first mammogram. What's it like?"

"It's like nothing you've done before!"

We laughed a lot about what we were doing, and then proceeded to the Imaging Center.

The Center had allowed me to come in early so I could decorate the room with brightly colored helium-filled balloons, all pink. A celebration cake, plates, forks, and napkins were in placed in the center of the table, surrounded by party sacks full of noise-makers, tiaras, chocolate, and game cards.

Each guest was given a party sack as they took their place around the table. We opened them together and pulled the contents out in front of us. A tiara! That was most important thing in the sack for we were to be royalty for the day. We were going to be the MammySlammy Queens!

The tiaras were made of shiny plastic decorated with huge impressive chunks of colored plastic gems. A few even had pink fluff on them. We stuck them in our hair rather than around our heads to avoid the headache that comes from scrunching lady-sized heads into adornments made for three year olds.

Chocolate was in abundance as we decided it is a necessity of life for royalty and really smart women. And we knew we were highly intelligent, or we wouldn't be here preserving our health. Of course, we ignored that chocolate might not be considered health food in some circles. In our circle, on that day, it was.

Noise-makers were fun for a moment, but a room full of laughing women can easily out do any noise maker.

Then, one of us (me) was summoned for the dreaded test. Insert drum roll here. I walked with a lot of to-do and bravado out the door, down the hall, and into the dressing room where I was asked to remove all clothing above the waist and put on a hospital-type cape that completely covered me. It tied in front so it could be easily opened for the mammogram.

A second person was invited to take the long walk to the dressing room and undress and drape herself while I was having my exam. Then another, and another, all taking their turn as we streamed in, one at a time.

One at a time, we had our mammogram, redressed ourselves, and reentered the party room where we played games and waited for the return of our friends, one at a time, to continue her participation in the ongoing party.

Each person received cheers of congratulations as she returned from her mammogram—alive, undamaged, and victorious.

"That wasn't so bad."

"It wasn't what I expected."

"I'd do it again…in a year."

"Hurray! I'm now an upper body contortionist!"

"At least you've got something to put on the x-ray plate. My goose bumps are now pressed folds."

We laughed a lot, deep belly laughs that exercise the whole body and release all the good endorphins. It was a joyful experience.

When everyone had their mammogram, we exchanged gifts. The gifts were all wonderful, fun, funny, and heartfelt. No one had any guidelines for what the gifts should be. Each was left to her own imagination. The gifts ranged from a bra that had the cups replaced with long, flat lacy socks. Another was a bag of pancake mix, hot pads, pancake turner and syrup. Yet another was a beautiful needle-point pillow that said 'Attitude'. Each gift was absolutely perfect.

We hated the day to end. We had shared stories, told jokes, played games, laughed hard, and bonded well. We hugged goodbye, vowing to make it a yearly event. We made sure everyone, including the staff at the Imaging Center, took a balloon home with them.

Some of us had joked for years that we would someday get a tattoo. We would talk about it, laugh about it, and forget about it for a while, and then the subject would surface again. We had 'talked the talk' for years, but had never 'walked the walk'. Now, it seemed it was time to stop the talking and do some walking. I don't know if any one of us *really* wanted a tattoo, but getting a tattoo seemed to make as much sense as making a party out of a mammogram. In fact, it became most important to really do it. So, off we went to the tattoo artist to get a tat to celebrate the occasion.

We moms and grandmothers entered a world previously unknown to us. The tattoo parlor artists were rather surprised to see us, but were very accommodating to us despite their obvious amusement of dealing with a bunch of women who were more mature than the usual clientele they work with. I'm sure they thought we were there looking for our naughty children or grandchildren.

We were obviously not well versed in how to get a tattoo. We looked through book after book, looking for the perfect tattoo. Somehow or other the skulls, crossbones, fire breathing dragons, motorcycles, and hearts with flowers didn't appeal to us.

Kay finally got brave and asked, "do you have any cartoons?"

And, they did.

We made our selections and then were invited to, one at a time, go with the artist in to another room. Now, we may have survived going in one at a time for a mammogram, but there was no way we were going to be isolated in a room alone with anyone wielding a needle of any kind. We all crammed into the tattoo room together where we supervised the process. There we were, piled on a couch, in chairs, on the floor, all over the place, and we were having one heck of a good time.

"Does it hurt?"

"Now what are you doing?"

"That is sooo cute!"

"Does Ellis know you are getting a tattoo?"

"Eeeek. He'll have a stroke!"

When we entered the tattoo parlor—(is it called a parlor?)—there were only a few teenage gang-wanna-be' kids, the artists who did the tattooing, and a few of their grown-up friends. The kids left as soon as they could get out the door when we came in. I guess they were nervous that we might know, and tell, their parents. Who knows? Anyway, when we were through being tattooed, had oooo'd and ahhhhh'd over one another's tattoo, had paid, and were ready to leave, we could hardly get through the crowd that had gathered in the entry room of the parlor. There had to have been a lot of phone calls made to get that many people down there so quickly to see the bunch of old ladies who were getting tattoos.

For us, it had been a daring adventure and we felt a sick sense of pride as we left with our newly penned declarations of life. We had little tattoos of comic book ducks, road-runners, Tweety Birds, peace frogs, and even some of the more gentle Celtic designs discreetly decorating parts of the body. We were 'women of the modern world', bravely declaring that life was fun and we were going to keep it that way.

We really had fun getting the tattoos and even more trying to decide exactly why we did it. We didn't just think outside of the box that night; we jumped out of the box, stomped the box flat, and then lit it on fire. Whoa, we were alive and doing well. We laughed our way to a restaurant for a late dinner before we all headed out in separate directions to our homes.

# Year 2: The number grew

During the year following our first big MammySlammy, we told others about the party and the fun we had participating, and the wonderful new friends we all made. Word of the hot new party was spreading. As people heard us talking and laughing about it, they asked how they could be included. Was it by special invitation? Did they have to join a club or something? Or, was it a special clique of friends? Would they be intruding? We were amazed, at first, and then we remembered that we weren't the only ones who hated to go for a mammogram alone.

No, we weren't a clique. There was no club and no special qualifying invitations. Anyone, and everyone, who wanted to participate was invited.

I must confess that there were a few women who just looked at us like we were totally out of our minds. I mean, why would getting a mammogram be fun? Sick! Get real! Normal women do not talk about breast examinations in concert with a party. Decent women simply refer to it as 'a yearly checkup' (which most do not do annually). We ignored their taunts and rolling of their eyes for we were women warriors with more to battle than their petty jibes. We were now actively engaged in a battle of never having another cancer story to tell. We were invincible! We invited them to attend the next party, but were not surprised that they chose not to participate.

A date for the second annual MammySlammy was selected, and those who had asked to attend were issued an invitation. They were asked to bring a friend with them. Believe it or not, most were excited not only to be invited, but to know they could extend the invitation to another friend. And, they came.

Once again, the Imagining Center was supportive in having us hold the party there. I decorated with balloons, which have become a must for our party. We love them, we buy them, we decorate with them, and we take them home.

We met for lunch, which was, and is, a good ice-breaker for meeting the new friends who had been added to the party. The second year we watched movies—"chick flicks"—and played cards using Maxine cards. We got so busy reading Maxine quotes and laughing that we often forgot where we were in the game.

We cheered as each was called in to the dressing room. Each was greeted with applause as she returned from the mammogram. And, when everyone was through, we had each person select and open a gift. We were a little more solemn this year. I'm sure it was because we each, independently, realized the importance of bonding together to make an unpleasant exam a wonderful experience. We seemed to realize the strength that comes from giving support to and caring for one another. We were beginning to see the importance of friendship and bonding. We were witnessing how reaching out to, and caring for others, returns benefits to our own lives. We had formed a sisterhood that could, and should, reach across the nation. We were women helping other women and rejoicing in how easy life could be if we were always there for one another. It was a comforting feeling that we discussed at great length over an evening salad.

# Year 3: More attending and even publicity

Many of us who were attending the MammySlammys were now actively involved in the Relay for Life Cancer Walk-a-thon, so we decided to do both the Slammy and the walk on the same day. This, we learned, was a great idea for those who are in their twenties, but we were a few years older than that. Partying all day, setting up our camps at the Relay for Life Walk-a-thon, and walking all night turned out to be more exhausting than necessary. Remember, we are moms and grandmothers! We plan to continue participating in both activities, just not the same day.

Once again, we had balloons. Only this year, the balloons were red, white, and blue. We had, as a country, watched an unreasonable attack on our nation and way of life. September 11th had been burned forever into our memories. How could someone do such a gross, horrible thing? Although pink ribbons and balloons are thought to be more appropriate for breast cancer activities, we felt the red, white, and blue were more appropriate this time. We were American women who were joined to fight cancer, in a country where we can gather at will without fear. We were not only declaring war on breast cancer, but on any foe who threatened the freedoms we enjoy.

Once again, each attendee was cheered as she left the room for her x-ray and, as she returned, was given a name of courage for completing her exam with bravery.

Channel 8 News heard about the MammySlammy and sent their camera and interviewer to our party. Who were these weird women, anyway? What a news story! The interview went well, and it was nicely edited. It stressed the importance of yearly mammograms in the detection of cancer, as well as the importance of caring for self and others. Thank you, Ysabel and Channel 8, for the coverage and especially for making us all look fifteen pounds lighter on television. Oh yes, we have invited the women who are employed at Channel 8 to participate in next year's celebration.

After the MammySlammy, we went to Ravsten Field in Idaho Falls to participate in the Relay for Life activity that is held yearly to earn money for the local American Cancer Society. It is a marvelous event in which to participate. We had two teams in the event: the Ya Ya Yo Yo's Team and the Cookies for Cancer Team. We built our campsites side by side, so we could get some serious visiting done. There were so many activities that it didn't leave too much time for chatting. We were so proud of our teams. We may not have been among the fastest movers, but we were definitely steady. We kept someone moving around the track from 7:00 P.M. until 7:00 A.M. (Way to go, Yo Yo's and Cookies!). We also had on-going fundraisers during the entire event. We sold cookies and other baked goods. One friend, Neal, brought his miniature horses and wagon and gave rides. We also had a dunking booth, which is always a good moneymaker. It was a wonderful event and our teams were absolutely awesome!

How does the Relay event work? Well, each team is made up of at least 10–13 people who are willing to earn at least $100 per team member plus pay the team registration fee. We weren't at all sure how we would raise the money, but we did it. Businesses were wonderful to donate items for auction or to sponsor team members. We became very skilled at seeking out resources.

One of the fund raisers was the selling of luminaries, a white paper bag that the purchaser could decorate with the name, picture, or token of remembrance for a loved one or friend that was currently dealing with cancer or who had survived, or died from, cancer. The luminaries were filled with dirt and a candle, which would be lit in a ceremony later that evening. The luminaries were placed around the track to provide light for the nighttime walkers.

Businesses from Idaho Falls and the surrounding areas kindly donated not only monetary donations, but also food, pop, water, etc. for the event. (Be sure to visit the wonderful business establishments in Idaho Falls, Blackfoot, Rexburg, and St. Anthony who so willingly give to make this event successful. The upper Snake River area proudly boasts that we have the friendliest and most caring communities that exist anywhere. Come and see for yourself!)

Each participant in the Relay was given a white Relay for Life tee shirt, and each cancer survivor on the team was given a different colored tee shirt that identified them as Cancer Survivors. The Relay kicks off with a gathering on the green as all the teams are introduced and the rules and procedures are explained. Teams are responsible to place all their luminary bags around the track.

The first lap of the evening was for those who have survived cancer. At 7:00 p.m., the daily temperature still registered hot. But a cool, refreshing summer breeze began the same time as the Survivor Walk. Many people, dressed in rich purple tee shirts, walked around the track, holding a purple balloon in hand. Some were bald from medication. Some were old, some young. Some were supported by others to ensure their walk could be finished successfully. Some were in wheelchairs or were using walkers. Some were recent survivors, some were veterans. But all walked proudly, knowing they had fought a good fight. It was so thrilling to participate in that first walk. At the end of the lap, all the purple balloons were released to the skies, accompanied by loud cheering and applause. Tears of joy flowed, as thankfulness leaked from the hearts of many.

The next lap added the caregivers and those who supported the cancer victims—doctors, oncologists, radiologists, phlebotomists, surgeons, nurses, CNAs, hospice staff, etc. Then family members and friends joined in the walk.

The rest of the evening was spent celebrating with music, pizza, pop, candy, fundraisers, and many, many activities, games, and healthy competitions…and, continuous walking or running.

Prizes were to be awarded to teams for best campsite theme, best team spirit, most participation, and various other things, including a prize to the team who made the most laps. Naturally, we 'non-kids' weren't too concerned with winning the prize for laps, especially when one of the high schools had entered a team of their cross-country runners. Wow, those kids were fast, enduring, and hardy. One would run for an hour or so, and then let another take his or her place to run for another hour or so, and so on and so on. We were all very proud of them as they repeatedly made a dozen or more laps to our one. Their energy and willingness to participate made us even more determined to keep walking, slow and steady as we were. I, personally, think it was a good thing for them to watch us so they will be better prepared when it is their turn to take their place in the aging population. We were heard to call out, "Go for it" as they came along side, and then as they passed by we would mutter, "I remember when…" Oh sure, we do. We were all star athletes, weren't we?

The darkness of night, ten o'clock, brought the time for the lighting of the luminaries. Once all the candles were lit, everyone was invited to walk together around the track. Hand in hand, heart to heart, people united in a common cause walked around the track, stopping now and then to read and admire a specific luminary.

They walked in support of those who currently were being treated for cancer.

"Stay well, Katie."

"Hang in there, Beryl."

"You can do it, Steve!"

They walked in appreciation for those who were survivors.

"Proud of you, Bobbe."

"Way to go, Sara."

"Tom, I didn't know you had cancer."

"A ten year survivor? Wonderful!"

"Remember to take time to play, Jim."

And on and on it went.

They walked all afternoon and night in memory of those who had not survived.

"There's the luminary Kathy made for her sister."

"That one is for my grandfather."

"Here's the one I made for Darrell."

"Hey, Jim, do you remember when we…?"

They walked with prayers in their hearts that the families and friends who had lost loved ones would be comforted.

"Help them accept and go on."

"Keep them safe."

They prayed for health and well-being. They walked with the hope that a cure will soon be found, not only for cancer, but for all the dark diseases that humanity faces everyday.

Walking the track lit by the glow of the luminaries throughout the darkness of night and in the early hours of morning became a hauntingly endearing time. For many, it was a time for healing and for peaceful remembering. As we walked and read the messages and names on the luminaries, we experienced a gentle calmness of knowing the appreciative value of friendship, of life, and of love for one another.

At 7:00 a.m., the final walk was announced. All the teams joined together for the last walk of the Relay. It was a walk of a unified team, resolving to return the next year, stronger and more determined. After the last walk, we gathered on the green for the closing ceremony. The beautiful voice of Katie, a high school student from Blackfoot who was recovering from Dysgerminoma—a rare form of cancer—began an a cappella rendition of the national anthem.

*"Oh, say, can you see, by the dawn's early light."*

Her hair was just now beginning to grow in and it framed her pixie face and beautiful eyes perfectly. Her voice was so strong and clear and angel-like that people were too stunned to stand. It was a voice that all the world should hear.

*"What so proudly we hailed at the twilight's last gleaming."*

People slowly rose to their feet, hats in hand and hands on hearts, as Katie's voice filled us with a newfound pride in country, in opportunity and accomplishment, and in self.

*"Oh! Thus be it ever,*
*when freemen shall stand*
*Between their loved homes*
*and the war's desolation!*
*Blest with victory and peace,*
*May the heaven-rescued land*
*Praise the Power that hath made and*
*preserved us a nation.*
*Then conquer we must,*
*for our cause it is just,*
*And this be our motto:*
*'In God is our trust.'*
*And the star-spangled banner*
*forever shall wave*
*O'er the land of the free*
*and the home of the brave!"*

The song ended. Silence hung for a brief moment as the audience caught their breath, and then applause and cheers filled the air. Katie left the stage. Tears of gratitude were wiped away as we returned to our assigned campsites, and packed them up into cars, vans, and trucks. We hugged and said our goodbyes and made our sleepy ways home, proud that we had the opportunity to participate in something so very, very wonderful.

With the warm glow of this MammySlammy Day and participation in the Relay for Life settling around me, I looked back at the long journey that began with my first mammogram.

# My
# Story

# Discovering

## January 31st

Cold shivers shook my body. My stomach knotted and pitched, turning the shivers into sobs. It can't be. Yes, it is a lump. Lumps are just harmless cysts, I told myself. No, I knew what it was. It was a good-sized lump. I quickly checked under my armpit. It felt lumpy too. By this time everything seemed to be lumps and bumps. The shower turned from gentle wafts of warm water to a torrential wounding and pounding force of water. My skin crawled and began to hurt. My head was spinning. I was crying, sobbing. I knew in my heart that it was cancer. No, it wasn't diagnosed yet, but it was a surety I couldn't deny. "Dear God no," I silently begged, "not now, not now. The girls need me. And, Dick? How will I tell Dick?"

I would turn forty-years-old in a few days. I was married, and mother of two daughters who were in the process of surviving teenage hormone-hell when I discovered, through BSE (breast self-examination), a lump in my breast. Dick, had retired from a career in the U S Navy, and we were settling into a civilian-styled life in Pocatello, Idaho. As the military moved us from state to state and country to country, we focused on someday returning to Pocatello, Idaho to settle down for the remainder of our lives. We had dreams and plans that centered there. I'd work or open a business and Dick would complete his education at Idaho State University. The girls would live in one place for their entire high school years, and would have good friends who wouldn't be moving when fathers were transferred. We would happily live in one place after dedicating twenty years to the defense of our great nation. Everything was supposed to be smooth sailing now that we were home. We had just bought the house on Alameda Avenue and were all happily and actively involved in our new style of life. This could not be happening to us now.

The shower water was turning cold. I realized I had been standing there staring at the shower walls, frozen in time, waiting for the lump to go away. I stopped crying, turned the water off, wrapped up in a towel, and made my way to the bedroom. Moving quietly, I shut the door. I needed to pull myself together before I said it aloud to anyone. I did not trust my voice to speak it aloud right now. I knew if I tried, my voice would crack, and I would start to cry with no guarantee of regaining composure. I checked for the lump again. It was still there. I guess I expected the lump to have dissolved because I wished it to be so, but it hadn't. I slipped into a nightgown, blew my hair dry, and checked again. Still there.

The girls were in the family room shooting pool and bantering back and forth. Dick was watching TV. I sat down by him and said, "I found a lump when I was showering; and, I'm afraid it could be…"

"Where?"

"My left breast."

Silence momentarily hung between us. His face turned ashen and his voice sounded shaken and unsure. "It could be a million things, Honey," he said. "But…"

"I will. I'll call a doctor in the morning. Let's not worry yet."

We spent the rest of the long night assuring each other that it would be okay.

We tossed and turned in bed. A cold winter wind blew fitfully as if to accompany our restlessness. Friday morning came slowly.

# February 1<sup>st</sup>

*I need to paint the bedroom,* I thought as I lay there waiting for the alarm to sound. I could hear birds singing as they sought food in the late winter offerings of the Russian-olive tree in our backyard. *We should take that tree out, too. It is so big and dirty and sends our allergies haywire, but the birds love it, and I enjoy their singing.* I checked the clock. It was still too early to get up.

Dick rolled over. "Are you awake?" he asked. I nodded. He put his arm around me and pulled me close to his side and said "It will be fine." I turned my face to his shoulder and cried. The alarm finally announced the official start of the day.

Noise. Lots of morning noise makes everything seem normal. Water sounds from the showers, hair dryers, opening and closing of closet doors, kids singing with the radio, dog needing out and in and out again, and TV news giving the state of the world today.

"Where's my hairdryer?"

"What's for breakfast?"

"I can't find my homework!"

Yes, lots of normal wonderful noise that on this day was especially treasured. The clatter and chatter of a normal day sounded like the most joyful of all symphonies. The front door slammed shut as Leisl and Melissa ran off to their day at school.

"Hon, I'm not going into class today," Dick said.

"Dick, please keep this as normal of a day as possible. If you stay here, we'll drive each other nuts! Call me later and I'll let you know when my appointment will be. OK?"

"Are you sure?" he asked.

"I am positive. It will give me time to get an appointment and get a few things done. I'll call the doctor at nine, so give me a call after your first class."

"But, Sharon…"

"Don't crowd me! I need some time to myself. Give me some space! Okay?" I snapped. I needed to blame someone for what I was going through. He didn't deserve any blame, but he was the only one there. We stared at each other across an angry wall of exclusion. He looked shocked, wounded. I knew I had been cruel. Nervousness and stress often make us into self-centered monsters, concerned only with our own needs.

*Hadn't I followed him around the world, handling things when he was gone? And wasn't he always gone? Good grief, he wasn't even there when Melissa was born. I was all alone. I had no husband there to hold my hand, to bring me flowers, or to hold our child while looking at me with his eyes full of love for his family. I was either left behind while his ship was out, or expected to move the girls, the dog, and me when school was out or when housing was available. I took care of the girls, the schooling, the finances and daily occurrences. I was there when they were ill, when they cried because their daddy was gone. I comforted them, kept them from harm. I took care of them and of me. I could handle any problem alone. And here he is now, crowding me. Pushing me. Wanting to make it all better. If I let him inside my fear, will he have to leave again? I need him. I need his assurances. I need him to hold me and tell me he'll never leave again for any reason.*

It was a brief moment of anger and self-pity. I had done well as a military wife. I had proven my strength through supporting his career. We had fun traveling to new places, having new opportunities and challenges. Life had its challenges and I—no, we—had handled them well. But now I felt I was fighting a singular war against inner panic and I needed to blame someone. I needed be able to deal with my own feelings and fear before I could consider his feelings. Somewhere in the unrealistic world of panic and worry, I knew if he went to the doctor with me it really would be cancer; and if I went alone, I would be just fine because he wouldn't be there to rescue me.

"Okay. I'll give you a call right after nine o'clock." Out he went, looking gray, tired and worried.

The house was quiet. Too quiet. It was only 7:30 a.m. and the doctor's office wouldn't answer calls until nine. Thank goodness I had already planned to stay home from work today. That saved giving others an explanation that I was not yet ready to make. I didn't want to tell anyone. I couldn't stand them looking at me as if I were wearing a death mask. I busied my self as best I could while the minutes dragged on and on.

# The Call

It was finally nine-o'clock.

"Hello. Doctor Horrocks' office. This is Jean. How may I help you?"

"Jean, this is Sharon Marler and I need to see the doctor today."

"Let me check. "Hmmmmm, the soonest we have an appointment is next week on Thursday at 3:00 p.m. Would that do?"

"No. I need to see him now. I...I...," and the tears choked my throat. "I found a lump in my left breast. It's a big lump. I'm sure it's nothing but..."

"Let me put you on hold for a minute, Sharon, and see what we can do."

Silence.

"Sharon, we can see you about ten o'clock. Can you make that?"

"I'll be there!"

The phone rang immediately as I hung it up from making the appointment. "Did you get an appointment?" Dick asked.

"Yes, at ten o'clock. But, Dick, let me go to this alone. If you come with, I'll be a bawl-baby and won't be able to even tell Horrocks what's wrong. Just meet me for lunch, okay?"

"Sharon, I think it would be better if I were there. You don't have to be alone in this. Include me."

"Dick, please, let me go alone. I can stay calmer if I don't have you there to rescue me. I need to do this."

"Fine," he said. "I'll see you at noon."

I knew I was shutting him out when I should be reaching out to him for help. I felt I had been conditioned by his twenty-years of military service to do things on my own. Besides, I justified, this was just for a check-up at this point of time. If it was nothing, I didn't want to appear to be over reactive. If it was cancer, I was prepared to handle it until I met him for lunch. More importantly, I knew we would have plenty of time to make decisions if the prognosis was bad.

# The visit to the Doctor

Dr. Horrocks' face grew somber as he checked the breast and armpit. He asked a number of questions and then said, "Let's get a mammogram taken and see what we are dealing with." He made a phone call and set up the appointment for the mammogram and blood work at the hospital that same day.

"The lab is ready for you as soon as you can get there, Sharon. Go get the x-rays and I'll call you at home as soon as I get the results. Don't worry, Sharon. We'll take care of it."

I was so encouraged. He had said not to worry so it must be just a cyst. The tests are just to confirm that it isn't cancer, I reasoned. I wished Dick was here with me. I loved him so and needed him there. I needed to smile at him and hear him say, "I told you everything would be okay." Why had I been so wicked and mean to him?!

I dressed and left the examination room to find Dick in the waiting room. I was so relieved to have him there, waiting, and *just being there* for me. I should have known he would be there. I smiled, sat down beside him, and calmly said, "Doctor Horrocks said not to worry. That's good news, huh? He said I needed to get a mammogram done today…right now, actually, and he'll call later with the results".

"Does he think it is serious?"

"He said not to worry. What do you think?"

We rushed to the lab, got the x-rays and blood work done and went to lunch.

Life was great, and the lunch was wonderful.

# The Phone Call

Dr. Horrocks called about 4:00 P.M. with the results of the tests.

"Sharon, it doesn't look good. It is definitely a tumor. We need a biopsy to determine if it is benign or malignant. I'd like you to see a surgeon. Who would you like to see?"

"Who can get me in the soonest?" I asked.

"I'll make some calls and get back with you."

Within a few minutes, Dr. Horrocks called to let me know I had an appointment with the surgeon on Monday morning at eleven o'clock. I looked at Dick. He knew.

"It was Dr. Horrocks", I said. "He wants me to see a surgeon Monday morning about a biopsy."

"It's just a precaution, Sharon. It will be alright, remember."

"I know."

Dick suggested we go to Sun Valley to spend the weekend. It would be wonderful to have a weekend away together in a beautiful location, and it should make time pass more quickly. We went, but it didn't work. Sun Valley was overcast and gray, and so were our spirits. We tried to put each other at ease with shaky conversation and weak laughter. It was no more than a shallow front to hide our worry behind.

# February 4<sup>th</sup>

I talked with the surgeon who advised me to check into the hospital the next day for tests and for an early Wednesday morning biopsy. He assured us it could be benign but added that we needed to move on it quickly for our peace of mind. We agreed.

Tumor. Benign. Malignant. New vocabulary used only in bad television soap operas. I could see Dr. Sven Jorgensen, the tall handsome sex-god doctor, telling the spoiled but beautiful heiress, Starry, that her life was going to end in spite of her father's money. 'Malignant, and rapidly growing', he would tell her. 'How long do I have?' Starry, the heiress, would ask. There she was with her full red lips pursed and huge blue eyes wide open, dampening with tears. The handsome hunk doctor would dramatically turn from her, stoop his shoulders, and say in a low, soft voice, 'weeks, Starry, only weeks.' She had to be courageous and withhold telling anyone she was going to die until this awful disease forced her to her bed. She would go for solitary walks along the shoreline, longing to be in the comforting arms of the war correspondent whom she had met and fallen deeply in love with only a few months ago. Then one day soon, she would be unable to rise from her bed. The family would call the handsome doctor to the mansion to care for her. Starry would slip into a coma, never confessing that she was pregnant with the child of that same war correspondent, the one who was married to her best friend.

Oh crap! This was not a soap opera. This was real life. My life. It was skiddilywampous, upside-down, and out of control. Panic crawled from the depths of my soul to my throat, choking and smothering me. *Be calm, Sharon*, I thought. *Stay calm.*

Monday evening we told Leisl and Melissa that I had to go in the hospital the next day. We assured them not to worry, and answered their questions as best we could. We told them we were sure everything would be fine. We knew Melissa believed us, but Leisl, who wore her feelings too exposed, had her doubts. Melissa gave me a hug, said she knew they (doctors) could fix it, and flitted off to find something else wonderful to do. Leisl dropped into her mothering role, and assured me that everything would be just fine. She went to her bedroom earlier than usual that night, and we gave her space to process her worries.

# Tuesday, February 5<sup>th</sup>

We got up early the next morning so I could make sure everything was done before checking into the hospital. I pulled the cover off the bird-cage and found the girls' parakeet lying on its back on the floor of the cage, legs out stiff and deader than the proverbial duck. We should have been upset, but we laughed about sick omens while Dick disposed of the poor dead thing, woke the girls, and told them about the bird. We hugged the girls, told them to have a good day, and told them that Dick would keep them informed of what was going on. They seemed to be doing okay, so we left for the hospital as they ran off to school.

I was nervous checking into the hospital, but I kept telling myself it was just for tests, an overnight stay, and an early morning biopsy. Don't panic, yet, I told myself over and over.

That evening, the surgeon entered the hospital room and closed the door behind him. He shook hands with Dick, looked at me and shook his head, and pulled a chair along side my bed.

"It doesn't look good. The x-rays show it is definitely a tumor. The tumor doesn't appear to be contained or cylinder in shape. It is uneven and has spidery growths or tendrils that strongly indicate cancer."

Dick slumped in his chair, his hands over his face. I struggled to find the words to answer the doctor. *Run, Sharon, run,* I thought. I looked toward Dick, then back at the doctor. I couldn't think. Words failed me. Dick stood up, took my hand, and said, "It'll be alright. It has to be."

"What can we expect?" I asked. "What do we do now?"

"We have several options. We can take you into surgery in the morning and do the biopsy, return you to your room to wait for the lab results, and schedule surgery for another day if it is, in fact, determined to be cancer. A second option is to keep you in the operating room until we get the report back from the lab. It won't take them long to get results. If the lab confirms it is cancer, we will determine if it is contained or if it has spread to the lymph nodes, and will proceed with whatever surgery is required to contain it. Do you need some time to decide what you want us to do?"

"Is there a chance it isn't cancer?"

"I wouldn't count on it, Sharon. The tests all indicate that there is a definite problem. I'll leave you two alone for a while so you can talk it over."

"No, don't go. I'd prefer to stay in the operating room until the lab confirms what it is. If surgery needs to be, just get it done. I don't want to be frightened twice."

Dick nodded his agreement.

"So be it," said the doctor. He said the nurse would come and take me to the education room to watch a video that would explain what would happen in the operating room, what I could expect, and choices I would have ahead of me.

The night was long. Words came hard while emotions ran the full gamut, some unspoken but understood between both of us. Emotional echoes pounded in the darkness of the unspoken words, words too frightening to speak. I asked Dick to go home and let Leisl and Melissa know what was happening. He didn't want to leave, but we both knew the girls needed him to be the one to tell them and to give them confidence that everything would be fine. I knew he needed time, and so did I. There was a lot of emotion to be processed separately before we could give support and understanding to each other.

Once told, both girls slipped into the *we-know-it-will-be-okay-daddy* role. They both assumed the role of caring for the house, the dog, themselves, and their dad. Their response to Dick was one of inner strength and faith that if their Dad said it would be alright, it would be. Before returning to the hospital, Dick called both sets of parents and let them know what was happening.

I was alone in the room. *"Please, God, don't let it be cancer. I don't want my life to end now,"* I prayed. *"I want to see grandchildren. I don't want to leave Dick. I want to stay here. Please, not now."* Tears stung my cheeks. My breath came in heaves of panic. My chest hurt, my arms moved in slow motion, and my legs felt like stone. I started to laugh as I thought, *wouldn't it be funny to die of a heart attack because I had cancer. Nothing like being scared to death!* The absurdity of it all was calming.

I was at peace when Dick returned, and he appeared to be so, too. Together is so important.

# Surgery and Healing

## February 6<sup>th</sup>—What a Freaky Way to Spend a Birthday

Sedated, dressed in a less-than-modest hospital gown and circle-cap, I traveled on a gurney to surgery. Sleepy. So sleepy, and soon…

"Can you hear me, Sharon? Talk to me. That's good."

"My feet are freezing."

"Get her another blanket."

My right hand reached toward the huge bandage on my chest.

"Sharon, we removed your left breast. It was in your lymph nodes, too. We're sure we got it all. Do you understand?"

Thick words from digitalized-figures hovering above me in a fog-filled room slowly penetrated reality, but did not have meaning. "Oh," was all I could say. I drifted back to where all was quiet and I could avoid reality for a little while longer. I slept.

Voices drifted around me during the day.

"I love you."

"You're doing fine."

"Just a sip."

"Roll up on your side. This shot will help."

"Let's sit up on the side of the bed. Just let your feet hang over the side. That's good. Now you can lie back down."

"Just sip it. You don't want to take in so much it makes you sick."

"How are you doing now?"

"This shot will help—roll up on your side."

"You're okay, Honey. They're sure they got it all. You'll be fine. I love you."

"Let's sit you up. There. That's better."

"Now you're getting warmer. That's good."

Silent apparitions floated in and out of the room. Some talked in muffled sounds; some just floated near the bed, re-arranging blankets, fluffing pillows, checking the bandage, offering medication, patting, cooing, and gently touching away the pain and fear.

"Sharon. We need to get you up so we can straighten your bed. Here. Let me help you. There you go. Just let your feet hang over the side. That's right. Now, lean on me and I'll help you sit down. Great. You're doing fine."

I was dizzy and weak. The bandage was bulky. Maybe it was just a biopsy and there was flesh beneath all the gauze. Yes, that's it. I'm going to be fine. It's just a little indentation in the breast, but nothing bad. The room is spinning. I need to lie down.

"Let's get back in bed now. There, that's better, isn't it? The doctor will be here in a few minutes. You're doing fine."

"You're doing great, Honey. The girls send their love."

I drifted back into the 'la-la' land of pain medication and rest.

# Recovering

Ethereal images haunt the nighttime hours in the hospital. Nurses magically appear to check vital signs and give soothing comfort and care. They fluff the pillows, straighten the bedding, whisper encouraging words of comfort and encouragement, and administer medicine to induce sleep and release from pain. Ghosts and angels float through the confusion of the mind, beckoning enticingly to those who are past a state of critically ill. Other apparitions of the mind and heart tug those who are less ill back to the reality of life. Dreams overcome the obvious, and the mind and body begin to heal. Daytime breaks out of the nighttime shadows, bringing new hopes and resolution. Okay, I tell myself, this is a little tough to face, but I think I can handle it. I'm strong. I'm resilient.

I found myself thinking back to the fourth grade in Salmon, Idaho. We studied Madame Marie Curie in school. I was fascinated that a woman would be involved in cancer research. I was unsure what cancer was but everyone spoke about it in hushed tones indicative that it was something very, very bad. I knew my father's sister, Myrtle, had cancer and everyone said she was going to die. She did. We were taught that Madame Curie's studies would save many lives. Her research eventually saved others, but it did not save her. She died.

Other thoughts haunted me: Was I going to live? Would my life make a difference? Would Dick and the girls love me even when they realized I was maimed? Scarred? What would I look like? It is rather difficult to be a D-size on the right-side of the body and a minus AAA on the other. I realized that my necklaces would never hang straight, not that they ever had. Would I look rumpled and crooked and…well, grotesque? Would I be an embarrassment to my family? Would Dick be able to hold me? Touch me? Love me? Make love to me?

Self-pity and humiliation filled the deepest depths of my soul-darkness. I knew Dick would stand by me, but wondered if it would be duty-bound or real. He doesn't deserve to be saddled with an ugly, misshapen hag, I thought. Tears leaked from the corners of my eyes. My chest, or what was left of my chest, ached with sadness.

"Good morning, Sweetness. How are you today?" Dick quickly moved across the room to my bedside and kissed me. "I love you," he said.

"Please close the door. I don't want people looking in here."

"Sharon, you…"

"Close the door. Please!"

"Sure."

A heavy quietness filled the room.

"You are so beautiful," he smiled as he spoke.

"Thanks."

Dick seated himself in the chair by the bed. "The girls are fine," he said. "They miss you and send their love. They'll be coming up this afternoon."

"I don't want them to see me like this," I said.

"No problem," he replied without addressing my self-pity and rude tone. "I brought you up a nightgown and your makeup. You'll have time to get ready."

Poor Dick, I thought. He doesn't get it. I don't want to scare them. I don't want them to see me like this…lop-sided and all. I don't want them to be repulsed by how I look. I don't want them to be ashamed of me.

"That's not what I meant!" I hurled at him. "Do you think they are ready to deal with me being so…Well, you know what I mean."

"They'll be just fine. You'll be just fine."

I calmed down and we visited until the nurse came in.

"Let's get you up and about," she said. "We'll get you bathed, into your own gown, and get your bed freshened. That will be nice, won't it? Here now, let me raise your bed and sit you up. Good job. Now, swing your legs over the side. Rest a minute. Now, just slide off the bed and into the chair. There. You're doing great."

The sponge bath felt so good. I brushed my hair back, and then was helped out of the rumpled hospital gown and into the one Dick had brought me. It was wonderful to have my own gown. It was soft, and felt like home. I tipped the mirror to where I could see more easily. I was pale. I put on a little makeup. Lipstick gave a little color. It seemed normal and non-freakish to be doing ordinary things.

"Wow," Dick said. "You look beautiful."

I smiled, really smiled. I felt human.

The clean bedding felt cool and crisp as I was helped back into bed. I was shaky and ready to rest. Breakfast was served…hot beef broth, soft-scrambled eggs, and Jell-o. What a treat! A few sips of broth and a bite or two of Jell-o was plenty.

I leaned back into the pillows and slept, while Dick slept sitting in a chair by the side of my bed. Things were going to get better.

# The Oncologist

"Good morning," he said. "I'm Dr. Ratcliffe. We'll be talking about some follow-up treatment."

The doctor, Dick and I talked about the options available. He said they had removed the breast and several lymph nodes and were sure they had taken care of all the cancer in that area. However, to ensure there were no stray cancer cells that could develop in other parts of the body, he recommended chemo therapy treatment. We agreed it would be the best option. The doctor said his office would set up a first appointment for me. He asked if we had questions, which we did not. It was so alien to us that we didn't know what to ask.

"Write out your questions as you think of them," he said. "I'll be back this evening and will be glad to answer them for you."

"Thank you, Dr. Ratcliffe. We will."

*Chemo therapy? That's the awful thing we see in movies where people with cancer poop and puke themselves to death. Their eyes look sunken. They are weak and pale. They do all this to gain a few months of life. This has to be a nightmare—a nightmare full of demons and sickening boogeymen that conspired to annihilate me from all I valued and loved. I wanted to wake up in Dick's arms and hear his reassuring, comforting words soothing away my fears. I couldn't believe this was happening to me.*

*Cancer! Chemo therapy! I wasn't the beautiful, dark-haired suffering Ali in Love Story. I wasn't Emma in Terms of Endearment. I was the red-haired me. I had a home, a husband, children, parents, and even a dog. There was no camera and it wasn't a story. It was real life. I was normal. I wanted to go home. I was so afraid I could feel my insides quaking.*

"He seems nice," I said.

"Yes, he does," said Dick. "He'll get us through this. You'll be fine."

Sure, I thought. Just like in the movies. In my best Ali-in-Love-Story-voice I said, "I love you, Dick."

He stayed by my side and I slept.

## Family, Dreams and Life

My dreams that afternoon centered on the girls. How I loved them!

Leisl Ann was born in Catania, Sicily, Italy while we were stationed at the U.S. Navy base, Sigonella. She was a little dark-haired baby, barely six pounds, with delicate features and a sweetness that one can only know as an emotion and cannot describe with words. She was gentle and comforting. When she smiled or laughed, the world responded. She grew up with music, dance, and with a genuine love for all living beings. She was, and is, a compassionate, intuitive, and truly a kind person. People could feel her genuine warmth and love for life and loved being around her.

Leisl always loved to sing. Her big voice from a little girl could be heard all over the neighborhood. She sang joyous songs praising everything wonderful in her world. When she was 18 months old, we left Sicily and returned home to the States. We were so thrilled to have our families meet our little songbird, Leisl, and to know that her sister would be welcomed to the world in Idaho.

Leisl and my father became quick friends. He would push her high in the swing while she sang, "there is sunshine in my eyes (eyes, not heart as the song was written) today" or "little lamb so white and fair" or any song she made up out of the sheer joy. She adored her Papa-Bear, as she had so named my dad.

She was now 16 years old, and had maintained and further refined her qualities, temperament, and personality. She couldn't stand to see others hurt or ill, so visiting the hospital was very difficult for her. I recognized the *I'm-panicky-but-being-adult-about-it* look, and knew she had to overcome a great deal of anxiety to enter my hospital room.

Melissa Rae was born shortly after we returned to Idaho from Sicily. Dick was stationed in Florida waiting for a ship and I was staying with my parents in Idaho when Melissa joined our family circle. She was three months old when Dick got to see her for the first time. Melissa was a cuddle-bug. We always called her *a drop of golden sun*. Everyone adored her. She was either into, on top of, underneath, or moving out of reach every minute of the day. She investigated life at breakneck speed.

It was so fun to watch baby Melissa copy-cat Leisl as she learned new skills and developed her own personality. She loved to dance. She would sing along with Leisl, and the two of them would twirl and spin until they got dizzy and fell down, and then they would both laugh as only children do.

Melissa gathered treasures, lost animals, but mostly pretty rocks. My dad loved to take her with him. He would scoop her up in his arms and off they would go, both wearing bib overalls, on a new adventure. They would return covered with black dust from gathering coal chips at the railroad switchyards, or covered with country-road dust and a pocket full of rocks from a mountain walk, or with fresh picked garden peas from the garden.

Melissa always loved to try new foods and to eat. Life, in general, was always an adventure, and she loved it so much she couldn't stop to think that life wouldn't go on forever. Now she was nearly fifteen. I couldn't believe they had grown up so fast.

"Mom?"

My eyes flew open and the loves of my life came to the bedside.

"You okay, mom?"

"I'm fine. Come on up here."

It was so good to see them. So normal. The joy of seeing them erased the self-pity I felt over how I looked and how frightened I was of what lay ahead for all of us.

The sterility of the hospital was forgotten as we hugged and visited. Leisl's shakiness subsided some. Still, she knew the severity of what was happening, and it showed in her every movement. She put on her best appearance and began to give me a run down on what was happening at home, how the house was being taken care of, and what she had fixed for Dick and Melissa to eat. She was a teen-ager forced into an adult role of providing care for the family. I told her I knew they would all do just fine. She relaxed a little, and it wasn't long before they both were sitting on the bed, laughing and talking. They filled my heart with the joy I needed.

Melissa began nibbling from my hospital tray.

"Mmmmmmmmm, Mom, this is good. Why didn't you eat it?"

I wondered where she put all the food in that skinny little body! She was so energetic and busy that she burned calories faster than she could eat them.

"This is a neat place, Mom. You have more tubes than freckles," she laughed. Sunshine spilled from her with every word. Her energy level far exceeded anything imaginable.

The girls rambled on about friends, activities, home life, and even told me that our dog, Aggie, missed me. They bantered about who really did clean the house—even Melissa's bedroom—and they promised they'd take care of their dad. They talked about the upcoming joint high school play, Lil Abner. Leisl was Mammy Yokum, and their friend Mike was Pappy Yokum, and…on and on.

"Will you be there, Mom?" Leisl asked. *How could I not be there*, I thought.

"I wouldn't miss it! I might not get there for every performance, but I'll be there…at least for the closing night. I promise."

Their visit was a reminder of how very much I had to live for. Dick was my heart, my soul, and my love. Leisl and Melissa were our joy, our beautiful daughters.

*Dear God, thank you for letting me share their lives. Please don't let it end now. I will do whatever is asked of me, but please don't let my life run out now. I need to be here. I have more to do. I can't go now. I won't go now. I belong here, with them. I will get well. I will.*

We talked more, hugged and kissed goodbye until the next visit, and off they went.

"They're a hoot!" I said to Dick.

"Yes, they are! Sharon, I know you're determined to make the play, but don't get your heart set on it. It might be too soon to be out and about."

"Oh, don't worry, I'll do whatever the doctor says. I promise."

I became stronger, more aware and coherent every day. I refused to dwell any longer on what had happened. I knew I had to concentrate on healing and accepting. Instead, I put my efforts into healing and ignoring. It was easier.

I smiled, was philosophical, and said all the right things to family and friends. I grew stronger. I refused to look at the ugly gash across the left side of my chest and under my left arm. I convinced myself that it wasn't important to look at it. I was alive and that was all that mattered.

"When can I go home?" I asked the doctor.

"You can go home when you are stronger. It should be a few more days. We need to make sure all your body functions are healthy. You need to get up and walk around, eat, drink and eliminate fluid, and…"

"I have to go to my daughters' play."

"We'll have to see how you are."

"I have to go. I promised. I'll be well enough to go, I know!"

The healing-war began and I resolved to be the victor. I ate well, drank a lot, walked miles in the hospital hallway, slept when I should, talked with the lady volunteer from the Cancer Society, and was cheerful.

My insides constantly churned and my mind imagined, but I suppressed the fears, the questions, the worries and I was happy—cheerful. Always cheerful. It was healthy to be cheerful. Cheerful meant I had a healthy body and a positive attitude. I was fine. Reality was placed on the back burner of the mind. I needed to go home.

The medical staff were amazed I was doing so well. The doctors said I was remarkable. I had such a healthy attitude and had built strength so quickly that I went home on Tuesday. I had about two weeks to build enough stamina to go to the play.

"Don't overdo," the doctor cautioned.

The next ten days were filled with daily trips to the hospital where the wound was cleaned and new dressing was applied. It appeared to be healing nicely. I exercised my arm and forced myself to do everything I possibly could with my left hand to keep the muscles from drawing up. It hurt to do the exercises, but I was determined to get 'normal' as quickly as possible. Outwardly, I smiled a lot and laughed hard, enjoying life to its fullest. Inside, I felt a growing anger and frustration.

I was tired of fighting to keep the cotton-blob-bra where it was supposed to be. It just wouldn't stay where it was supposed to. If I reached for something, it would crawl toward my chin. After some thought, I decided to pin a ribbon to both my bra and the waistband of my slacks. All that did was jack the pants up in front, which looked awful and felt weird. Ribbon didn't allow for movement.

Something had to work! I decided to try a piece of elastic. It should stretch when I reached or moved, and should retract back in place when I relaxed. That was how it *should* work, not how it *did* work. The pants still hitched up in front, just with more of a spring action. I'd pull the pants back down in place and the shirt would pull with it making me look a lot like Quasimodo. It was difficult but possible to look comfortable, poised, and in control when sitting or standing, but walking was a whole new experience! Step, pants jump up, pull pants down, shirt pulls down, pull shirt up and pants spring alive, step, pants spring up, stumble, shirt pulls askew, pants pull down and then spring up. You get the idea, I'm sure! It was more like limerick-run-amok than poetry-in-motion. I thought about buying a big red clown nose and a pair of black glass frames with a mustache attached to wear with my left breast-blob under my chin, jumping pants and a Quasimodo-style shirt. I constantly reminded myself that I needed to quit worrying about appearance over substance and simply be glad I was alive.

We attended some of the dress rehearsal of the play. I got tired too quickly so we didn't stay for all of it. I missed opening night, and the Friday night performance but Saturday was closing night and I was going come hell or high water.

The auditorium was packed. Dick held my arm and guided me to seats reserved for us in the front section of the auditorium. I knew we had the most talented daughters in the world. I was so proud of them.

Halfway through the play I started feeling weak, tired and dizzy. I clutched the arms of the chair to remain upright. Sweat poured down my back between my shoulder blades. The cotton-stuffed left-side of my bra kept crawling up my front, feeling like it was jammed under my chin in an effort to block my air passages. I tried to be discreet in pushing it back in its place. It was hot. I was having difficulty breathing.

Applause from the audience made my mind and body throb. Curtain calls. A wonderful play. Talented daughter. Final bows. We were on our feet applauding. The curtain opened and the cast welcomed the audience on the stage for hugs and congratulations. I made it to the stage. I hugged Leisl and her friends. Good job, kids. Clammy. Good acting. Good directing. Great job. The room was swimming. I couldn't see the stairs leading down from the stage. Melissa had noticed me having difficulty.

"Are you alright, Mom?"

"No, help me down from the stage."

Melissa guided me down the stairs. The room was spinning and pitching. Dick appeared through the haze and helped me back to my chair. Sick. So sick. I felt weak and shaky. Dick assured me I was just overtired. When the crowd thinned enough to make our way out of the building, I dizzily let Dick lead me to the car. My stomach hurt. My head was spinning. I felt sticky hot. My insides churned. Dizzy. I leaned back into the car seat. I felt I had entered the twilight zone of melting away.

# The Choice

Dick all but carried me into the house. I made it to the bathroom. I was vomiting. My stomach was cramping. I had a fever. Diarrhea hit violently. Dick called the hospital, and they called the surgeon who had done the surgery. The surgeon prescribed Compazine and told Dick where he could get it filled. I took the recommended dose. I threw it up. The diarrhea and vomiting continued. I grew weaker. Dick put in another call to the doctor. He said to take more of the medication since I had vomited it up. Hesitatingly, Dick administered another dose. I was too weak to get out of bed. Dick put a towel under me so I wouldn't soil the bed, and put a pail by the side of the bed to catch the vomit. The doctor said the medicine would kick in soon and a good night's rest was all that was needed.

Sunday came and I grew weaker. The vomiting had turned to dry heaves. I was freezing cold despite the mound of quilts piled on me. By nighttime, I was too weak to speak. Dick called the surgeon again and was told to have me come into the office Monday morning. Dick shouted into the phone that if I didn't get help, I wouldn't be alive Monday morning. He slammed the phone down, gathered me up, put me in the car and took me to the hospital.

The emergency room staff brought a wheelchair to the car and rolled me into an examining room. The attending nurse took my blood pressure…twice. It was getting dangerously low. I had no control over my bowels or with controlling the vomiting. I curled up on the examining table too weak to respond. The surgeon was contacted. He told the nurse to administer a large dose of Demerol. She argued with him over the amount prescribed. He lessened the amount a little. She asked him to please come in and exam me. He said he would see me first thing in the morning and ordered her to give me what he had prescribed.

She gave me the injection as instructed. I had soiled my gown so she helped me into another. I felt entirely helpless. I had no strength to fight off the death that seemed to be lurking. I was too dehydrated and weak to even care. I fell asleep. The nurse advised Dick to go home with the girls and get some rest. She told him I would rest, and if I wakened or if there were problems, she would call him.

The room was dark. Large balls of sand particles would fall toward me, splitting into drops of harmless micro streaks of light. The room would lurch and pitch in dizzying throws like a canoe riding out a tidal wave. Then, it stilled. A cool hand brushed my forehead. Someone took my arm. I felt movement and heard the words Code Blue, room something or other. Was it my room? I heard the sound of running feet. My bed turned into a magic carpet ride. It flew through the air while bodiless-feet quickly ran along side. I saw panels of colored light pass. Doors flew open and I entered into a cool darkness.

"Try again. We need to know what's going on."

"I can't find a vein."

"Try again."

"It's just not there. Blood pressure is falling."

"What is it?"

"Forty. Forty over doldrums."

"What?!"

"Forty high…nothing low."

"Her system is shutting down."

Voices turned into muffled sounds of *wah-mumph-snah-tszu* words of no meaning. I felt the entire scene of patient, doctors, machines, and bed shrinking away while I watched from the sidelines. I stood against the wall watching the pixilated medical staff work with my form lying on the bed. I stood next to a new friend-being, a Comforter, whose reassuring presence established a calm environment in the middle of chaos. No words were spoken aloud, but we conversed, exchanging words heard only between us. I knew I was supposed to go with this Being. I wanted to stay. I wanted to go. It would be easier to go than to stay.

"Dick's looking through the window. Why won't they let him come in?" I asked.

"Because they are trying to save your life. Family members often get in the way and make it difficult for them to do what is needed."

"They're good men." There was a length of quiet time as we watched them work. Then I asked, "Why is Doctor Horrocks crying?"

"He's tired. He has worked long and hard to save you. He has been a good friend to the Marler family for a long time. It is hard for him to lose you."

"There's my new doctor, the oncologist."

"Yes. They called him, too."

"What does he mean by 'should we call it'?"

"They aren't getting a heartbeat and they think you have passed on."

"Have I?"

"You know the answer."

"Look! There's Dr. Levin. I always liked him. He hasn't given up on me."

The angel-being Comforter chuckled and said, "he rarely gives up. He is so determined."

I laughed a little, too. "I know. He's quite the guy. I like him."

I looked around the room and then back towards Dick.

"Dick looks frightened and so sad."

"Of course he does. He doesn't want to lose you. But it is time to go."

"I know."

We turned and started to move away. I looked back at my body, my shell, on the bed. All the doctors stood in a circle with shoulders bent forward. They were weary, and had stopped working. The time seemed to be frozen in slow motion.

I let my eyes turn one more time towards Dick.

"I love you, Dick, with all my heart and soul."

His eyes were full of tears. He knew why the doctors had stopped working. The room was too quiet. The doctors slowly turned, looked at the clock, and then back at me. Dick's hand pushed against the window to lend him support.

Movement and sound seemed suspended in never-never land. It was quiet. Absolute silence. Deafening silence.

"I can't go," I said. "I can't do this. Please, let me stay."

"Are you sure?"

I was torn; I knew we would be going somewhere good. I knew I wouldn't be sick or hurt. I knew if I stayed, the years ahead would be difficult for all of us. I knew if I went, Dick and the girls would miss me and would be hurt, but I knew they would heal. I knew I needed to go.

Comforter was steps ahead of me, reaching back to take my hand. I reached out for his hand and we started to move forward. It was exhilarating to be going to something new and most pleasant.

Then I paused and looked back at Dick.

"I can't go without him. Not now. I have to stay. Please, please let me stay."

The Friend smiled. "It will be hard for you and everyone if you choose to stay. It will be easier if you come."

"I know, but I have to stay."

Are you willing to stay knowing how hard it will be for you? For everyone?"

"Yes, I know. I'm just not ready to go. I want to stay with Dick. I want to raise my daughters. I want to stay here with them."

The doctors slowly started to move away from my bed, removing their masks and gloves.

"Wait! She took a breath. Don't call it! Don't call it! Sharon…Sharon…It's Dr. Levin. If you can hear me, squeeze my hand. Concentrate, Sharon. Do it!"

I saw the Being dissolve into the dark. Our hearts and minds were no longer one. I could no longer connect with him, and I felt a deep empty sadness to have the Comforter take his leave.

My eyes fluttered open. I hurt. They were hurting me. My throat was dry and swollen. Tubes. Needles. Dizzy.

"I'm thirsty," I croaked.

"She's back." There was a brief pause and then a cheer from the doctors.

"Sharon, you're going to be okay."

"I'm thirsty."

"You can't have any water yet, Sharon. We're going to try one more time to get a blood test, Sharon. We're having trouble finding a good vein, so we have to try in the groin. OK?"

"Not 'til I get water. I'm thirsty."

"No water, Sharon."

"Ice?"

"Someone get some ice."

The ice appeared and Dr. Levin painted my lips with the ice. "That's the best we can do right now, Sharon."

"More. I want more."

"Alright, but don't swallow the water when it melts. Just suck on it, and spit the water out."

"Okay."

The ice felt so wonderfully refreshing. My dry mouth sucked in the cooling liquid like a sponge.

"Spit out the water, Sharon. Don't swallow."

"Want more."

"No, not now."

"Yes."

"Okay, just one more piece. There. Now can we try to get some blood?"

"Yes, if I can have more ice." They laughed.

I looked toward the window. Dick's head was bowed. I knew he realized I had come back. I was grateful for the One, my Friend and Comforter—whether he was real or imagined—who stood with me calmly watching life's transition to somewhere not of this earth, and back again. I knew he would return another time.

I started to feel warm again and I smiled with the happiness of knowing I would get well and go home. I drifted into a deep healing sleep.

# *Awakening*

Time is immeasurable when you are seriously ill. You sleep, respond to nursing care, walk when told, sleep some more, and start over. Days and nights intermingle, giving concentration to the healing process rather than to the illness. The focus is on healing and not on pain, appearance, or surroundings. Eventually, as the body gets stronger, you begin to want more. You want to smell fresh, outdoor air. You want your own gowns and slippers; in fact, you start wanting clothing and unrestricted movement. And you want real food—pizza, crisp salads with Buddy's dressing, tacos, and steamed vegetables with seasoning. You want crisp crackers and carrot sticks out of your own fridge. You want to pet your dog, sit on the lawn, and do all the wonderful things that confirmed you were alive and normal.

I noticed that the girls would always visit at mealtime. Melissa loved hospital food. She would bring little treats and trade me for what was on my food tray. Thank goodness Leisl had become more at ease with hospital visits. Parents visited for a few minutes nearly everyday. My friend, Roma, worked at the hospital and stopped at my room for a frequent cheery visit. My bishop and his wife visited once, but they stood in the hallway and awkwardly visited through the door opening. Punk (Norman), one of Dick's brothers, drove over from Boise and spent several days visiting. He even smuggled in a small pepperoni pizza one evening. It was so good!

There is a lot that could be said for being in the hospital for an extended time, but those experiences are so individualized that I choose not to talk further about it. Let me just say that getting well requires infinite patience from all concerned. Emotions, fatigue, medication, caring staff, loved ones, and personal determinations frame each day of

a hospital stay. The nursing staff and doctors treat the medical problems, but healing demands much more than medicine. It requires
immeasurable love and understanding from self and everyone.

The day finally came when I was strong enough to go home. I was
so excited I could barely contain the tears of joy. Dr. Ratcliffe talked
with Dick and me before my release from the hospital and explained
that he felt I was still too weak to begin chemo therapy.

"Let's give the surgical wound a little more time to heal and the
body to get stronger."

He handed me an appointment card with a time and date on it. "See
you in three weeks. I wish we could start sooner."

He had refreshed my health status with me. They had removed the
breast and lymph nodes and, hopefully, had contained the cancer. The
infection had taken a toll on my body; the incision was open and
would need to be cleaned and have the bandage changed twice a day. I
would continue on antibiotics for another two weeks. It would take
time for the incision to heal, and I would be unable to get a real prosthesis until it was healed entirely with healthy tissue. I would continue
to balance myself with a cotton stuffed bra.

"You are a fighter, Sharon, or you wouldn't be alive today. I want
you to beat this and I will do all I can to see you do."

After spending ten days in ICU, five days in CCU, and another
seven days in a regular room, I was going home. I was taken by wheelchair to the check-out desk where I was handed pieces of paper and a
pen. "Just sign here," the office staff said. I stared at the paper and at
the pen in my hand. I knew something should be happening, but nothing did. "Here, dear, just sign your name here."

I could not make anything happen. The paper was covered with
unreadable gobble-gook. It made no sense to write my name on the
line provided. And, just how did this *pen and name on paper* thing
work? I was getting panicky. I couldn't breathe and I was getting dizzy.
I knew I should be able to read and to write, but the process of how
just wasn't there.

"Dick, would you sign it for me? I'm too shaky." I managed to say.

"Sure, no problem."

*No problem I thought. I have dropped into an alien world where everyone but me could read and write, and there is no problem. I don't know what is going on. I can't tell people that I'm forty years old, lop-sided, and illiterate, too. Why is this happening? Stay calm, Sharon, this is just temporary. It will pass. It's just a fluke, not real at all. But it was.*

"You stay well," the hospital staff said as they helped me into the car. "Take care of yourself. Bye."

# Home

Words cannot describe how good it was to be in a car, being driven once-around-the-city, and eventually to my home. The yard was freshly mowed and trimmed, spring flowers were blooming, and everything looked vibrantly alive.

"Mom, we got the house cleaned for you!" Melissa shouted as she bounded toward the car with Leisl following close behind and *Aggie,* the dog, jumping and barking with excitement.

"Really Melissa, she knew we would!" said Leisl. "Do you need anything, Mom?"

"No, not a thing. Let's go in and just talk. It is so good to be home."

I loved our home on Alameda Avenue. The big fenced back yard had huge mature trees and a sense of calming quietude. The neighbor's dog, a big Labrador, would run to the fence for a greeting and a pat on the head. It was a silly old dog that loved to play with cinderblocks and tires, not exactly the usual doggie toys but he had fun with them. The big Russian Olive trees invited birds of all kinds to nest, and chirp and sing. The tiers of the yard were joined with a sloping ridge that was perfect to spread a blanket to lie on and bask in the lushness of it all.

The flower gardens under the windows in the front gave the feeling of home-ness. I was alive and well, and things would get better. We were a family and we were together.

The next few weeks were spent resting at home, going for long drives and short walks. Then, one day, while everyone was at school or work, I dressed myself, put on makeup, combed my hair, and ventured the four blocks to the shopping plaza. I was terrified to be going out in public without my protective family around me. I knew it had to be done someday, and this day was as good as any to see what would happen. I took my time walking to the store, wondering with every step if it was a good idea to be going alone.

*What if I see someone I know? Will people think I looked different, weird, and even ugly? Would the cotton-glob-boob stay in place? If they asked about my health, would they really want to know or would it be just the courteous thing for them to ask? Get a hold on this, Sharon. You're way off course. People aren't rude. They understand. Just go in the store and act normal. Good grief, it's a long way to walk! I should have waited for some-one to bring me here. No, you can do it. Just stay calm and move slowly. You'll do okay.*

I entered the store, grabbed a shopping cart, and pushed it down the aisle, totally enjoying the normalness of shopping. A store clerk asked if she could help me find something. "No, thank you. I just came to look." The sheer volume of items and the huge size of the store were disconcerting. It had been nearly two months since I had been in a store.

Then I saw a Carol, a member of our church congregation, coming toward me. "Sharon. I didn't expect to see you out and about," she said. "I should have come to visit, but I heard you were more dead than alive. I'm thrilled to see you doing so well."

"Thanks, Carol. It was pretty rough for a while, but I'm doing fine."

"I just can't believe you are out and about so soon. It must have been hard to do; I mean, you look so bad!"

"It wasn't easy, but I'm doing okay." *What does she mean by 'you look so bad'? I thought I looked all right. Wait. She was still talking. I needed to pay attention and listen to her.*

"I can't believe how strong your girls are, Sharon. They don't act at all embarrassed by how you look now. I'm not sure my daughter would be that brave if I'd had a mastectomy and looked so lopsided." I was so shocked I just stood there, looking at her and blinking. "Goodness, Sharon," she continued, "the Lord has given you such a strong spirit. I know you'll be just fine."

She hugged me, turned to move on, and then paused and asked as an after thought, "Do you need me to help you get your shopping done? I have a few minutes to spare."

"Excuse me," I said, as I turned and ran out of the store. I stumbled toward home, crying and gasping for air as the words "they don't act at all embarrassed by how you look now" rang in my ears. I made it to the security of my home, stood in front of a mirror, and pulled my shirt and the bandages off to look at the wound. It gaped open and looked horrendously ugly. It was so gross. I replaced the bandage, put on my shirt and added a sweatshirt to further hide my appearance. One more look in the mirror showed that my eyes were not only red from crying but were sunken and had dark circles under them. My hair was brittle and had lost vibrancy of color. I was pale, and yes, my cotton-stuffed-boob looked lumpy and had pulled uneven. I looked bloated, puffy and pasty. I was struggling to learn to read and write again. I was an ugly idiot who was an embarrassment to everyone. I crawled on the bed and sobbed myself to sleep.

I awoke to the smell of dinner being cooked. Wonderful smells of roast beef, potatoes, gravy, green beans, and fresh-baked bread wafted down the hallway and into the bedroom. I couldn't believe how hungry I was. Dick and the girls were busy setting the table, telling jokes and laughing. I forgot my bout of self-pity, brushed my hair in place, and went to join them.

"Well, good morning Sunshine. Glad you could make it for dinner. Did you have a good nap?"

"Yes. My goodness that smells good. When do we eat?"

"Right now. Have a seat."

It was delicious. As we ate and joked and laughed through dinner, I determined to end the trips to the pitty-potty and make things better. After the dishes were done, I asked the girls to help me update my makeup and hairstyle.

"What style, Mom? It's shot, ya' know?"

"Yes, I know. But see what you two can do with it."

"I think it's impossible, but we'll try," they teased. Out came the electric hair rollers, all their makeup, brushes, combs, and mirrors. Leisl curled my hair, and the two of them worked over my makeup.

"Wow, Mom, you actually look pretty good!" said Melissa. "In fact, you look beautiful!"

"You really do, Mom," echoed Leisl. "Daddy, come and look at Mom."

I looked in the mirror. I did look good and, more importantly, I felt great. We spent the evening watching a movie, eating popcorn and truly enjoying being together. No fronts. No fears. We were together, genuinely having fun.

When we went to bed that night, Dick pulled me close as he always did, told me he loved me, and kissed me goodnight. Then he kissed me again, and again. We had not shared intimacy since I had found the lump. I pulled away from him and told him goodnight. He waited a minute or two and then assured me that nothing had changed between us. Defensively, and fearfully, I told him he didn't need to make love to me out of obligation or pity. I could understand him being repulsed by how I looked. I couldn't stand to look at it, so why did I think he would be able to deal with it. I told him I appreciated his pretending nothing was different, but it was and if he wanted to leave, he could.

He remained quiet for a minute before he spoke. He told me he felt helpless because he couldn't make the cancer go away, he couldn't fix it. He said he knew I was very sad and very angry. He also told me that he was in love with me, not with just my breasts, nor my legs nor arms—just with me, and that he still found me to be sexy, and beautiful, and someone he wanted to spend the rest of his life with.

He took time with me, and gentled me back into a world of response and sexual satisfaction. He held me tightly in his arms all that night, and I felt secure and deeply loved for the first time in many weeks. I felt beautiful, self-confident, and ever so fortunate to have someone that loved me as a person, a whole person.

# Reality Really Does Bite

Reality of the high price of survival started being delivered each day by the mailman. We were deeply in debt. The labs, the doctors, the hospital costs were astronomical. We didn't have catastrophic insurance and we soon found that our insurance did not have a ceiling price on co-payment. We owed $168,000 over and above what the insurance had paid. Dick dropped out of school his last semester and accepted a job at the Youth Services Center in St. Anthony, Idaho. He borrowed a motor home from his parents and moved to St. Anthony, commuting home when time and money allowed. When he couldn't get home, I drove to St. Anthony to spend weekends with him. We put our house up for sale. Life had definitely changed for us. At least he was able to get open-enrollment insurance for all the family. That would help with the money for chemo therapy.

The incision was slow in healing. Instead of the anticipated three weeks, it took nearly six weeks. But at long last, it was healed and I could begin chemo and get a real prosthesis. No more chin-blobs for me!

# I like boobs-a-lot, or
# the day I got my prosthesis

The doctors had ruled out reconstructive surgery because of the high risk of infection, body weakness, and the chemo therapy. However, they all concurred I was healed enough to wear a prosthesis. I was elated. I thought I would just walk in and say, give me a left-sided D cup prosthesis and be done. There were many to choose from made from a variety of materials into several breast-like shapes and sold for varying prices. The fitting included a selection of bras that had pockets sewn in to hold the prosthesis. The most wonderful thing about all of the prosthesis forms was that they were weighted with a material that approximated the movement, feel, and weight of natural tissue. Hurray! At first the prosthesis seemed too heavy, but in time it began to feel natural. It provided the balance my body needed and, more importantly, didn't ride up under my chin!

Now, here is a real kicker for you. The insurance companies will provide prosthesis every couple of years for someone who has lost a leg or an arm. They realize that artificial body parts can wear out or changes in the body can occur that require adaptation to the artificial limb. However, insurance companies only pay for one breast prosthesis for mastectomy patients, no matter how long you live. Women, I assume, are not to lose or gain weight, change bra sizes, nor outlast their one and only fake breast. Now, let's add the icing on the cake. Keep your receipts because the cost of doctor prescribed breast forms and bras with pockets may be tax deductible, but only if the receipt is marked as medical expense. Isn't that just ducky? Who in the world would buy breast prosthesis or a weird pocketed bra for non-medical reasons? How bizarre! But, I was elated to have my clothing hang almost right for the first time in months and soon became accustomed to the weight and feel of the prosthesis. It felt great to look and feel semi-normal again.

# Chemo therapy 101

My first chemo therapy treatment was on April 26th at 3:30 p.m. Dr. Ratcliffe explained that I was a Class II Type cancer patient, meaning the cancer had spread from the breast to the lymph glands. He told me that chemo therapy should reach any errant cancer cells that were not contained or removed by surgery. No guarantees would be given, but the opportunity to increase the chance of survival was there, and I was ready to do whatever was required.

I would orally take Cytoxan (Cyclophosphamide) and Prednisone twice a day, as prescribed. Doctor Ratcliffe explained what each drug was for and what the side effects could be.

Cytoxan has a direct chemical interaction with the cells in that it stops or slows down cell growth. Possible side effects are nausea, vomiting, and depression of bone marrow, the blood-forming organ. The bone marrow, when depressed, leads to a depression of white cells (important for fighting infections), depression of blood platelets (important in blood clotting), and depression of red blood cells or hemoglobin (transfusion may be required to correct this). Other adverse effects that might be seen are hair loss, which is not permanent, and bleeding from the bladder due to a toxic cystitis of the bladder wall. Continued administration may lead to bladder contraction, amenorrhea and possible sterility.

The possible adverse effects of Prednisone are changes in physical appearance, namely in the form of increased weight and a puffy appearance, especially in the face. Rarely high blood pressure can occur or an increase in the sugar content of the blood. A common effect seen is a marked increase in appetite. In adults, this drug also may potentiate the formation of GI ulcers. Osteoporosis may occur in prolonged administration (demineralization of the bones).

Three other drugs—Vincristine, Methotrexate, and 5-Fluorouracil—would be administered intravenously once a week.

The possible adverse effects of Vincristine are hair loss that is not permanent, and local burns if this drug escapes the vein. It can affect the peripheral nerves in one of the extremities causing changes in some muscle action and muscle tone. Severe constipation can occur. Vincristine depresses the blood-forming organ, the bone marrow, mostly the red blood cells and this may require transfusion to correct.

Methotrexate can cause mouth lesions in the form of painful patches on the lips, gums, and mucosa of the mouth. These clear rapidly when the drug is discontinued. There can also occur ulceration of other parts of the digestive tract with abdominal pain, vomiting, and diarrhea. This drug can also depress the blood-forming organ, the bone marrow, which leads to a depression of white cells needed for fighting infections, the blood platelets needed for blood clotting, and red cells or hemoglobin that may require transfusion to correct.

5-Fluorouracil causes nausea, vomiting, sore mouth, diarrhea, skin rash, reversible hair loss, increased skin pigmentation, light sensitivity, and once again the depression of bone marrow. Another possible side effect, though rare, is uncoordinated gait.

With all that to look forward to, I was pretty nervous about my first chemo treatment. My body tingled with heat as the drugs were fed into the veins. It made my throat feel hot and dry and I experienced some nausea but nothing severe like I expected.

I slept well, but awoke the next morning to a violent episode of vomiting and diarrhea. It was uncomfortable, but manageable. My feet, legs, and hips ached and I experienced a great deal of fatigue and napped for a good 2–3 hours that day. That was all there was to it. Not a big thing to deal with.

Dick came home Friday night and we spent the weekend playing hard. We went fishing Saturday afternoon and had a marvelous time. Dick was fishing from a float tube while the girls and I used spinning rods from the bank. Leisl, Melissa and I refused to thread the worms on hooks, so Dick made up a bunch of snap-on leaders and baited the hooks for us. We'd catch a fish, warhoop and dance around in a victory dance, drop the fish in the creel, unsnap the leader, attach a new one, and catch another fish. An early spring breeze was blowing, the sun was warm, and we had a marvelous time. Dick snapped photographs of us holding our fish. It had been a long time since the four of us had this much fun and laughed this hard. We took the fish home, cooked them up with onions and potatoes, and enjoyed a delicious supper. It was a great day.

Dick returned to St. Anthony. The girls and I continued living in Pocatello, hoping the house would sell quickly so we could get out from under the immense pressure and stress our financial situation was causing.

The girls dropped the film off at the drugstore for processing and picked them up a few days later. They were thrilled with the photographs.

"Hey, look at this one, mom. You look gorgeous," said Melissa.

I took the photo and looked at it. My face looked like a big fat sickly-white balloon. My hair looked as dry as over-bleached, over-colored hair, and my skin looked green and dry. Why would Melissa say I looked beautiful? That was cruel. My entire body looked bloated and puffy. I freaked out and tore the photograph into pieces.

"Hey. Why did you do that? I wanted it," screamed Melissa.

"You can't have it," I screamed at her. "It's awful. I'm ugly. Ugly!" I threw it in the wastepaper basket, ran to my room, sobbing, and slammed the door. The words "I can't believe how strong your girls are, Sharon. They don't act at all embarrassed by how you look now," rang in my ears.

My head pounded with pain. I knew I had hurt Melissa. I so didn't want to do that, but I had. Seeing how I looked in a photograph made me ill. I wondered if Melissa would understand my reaction. She didn't. She thought I looked beautiful, probably because she felt it was the day we finally returned to a point of real life and living and laughing. And I had ruined the beauty of the day for her by overreacting to how I looked. I was ashamed and sickened by how I had acted. I apologized to her, hugged her, and told her I loved her but there was no way to mend the hurt. We both would just have to outlive that it happened.

# Life Goes On

The chemo therapy sessions, along with re-learning to read and write, made for an interesting year. Everything became a statistic, and time gained was always a goal. I heard 30% chance of survival, 50% reoccurrence, 40% of this and 20% of that. The chemicals weaken the body, the soul, and the mind. Familiar words disappear. You observe but don't record or retain. Decision-making becomes a joke. You can't make decisions if you can't think straight.

Chemo therapy chemicals affect your taste and smell. Foods taste metallic. I hated to call it therapy. Therapy should make one feel better. Chemo, however, is unpredictable. Symptoms vary. Sometimes it would affect my nervous system; my skin would crawl and I'd feel agitated and couldn't think. It would hurt to stand or sit or lie down. Another week's treatment would leave me fatigued and bone tired. One treatment would make me feel a little queasy but okay while another would leave me sicker than heck! Puking, pooping, and wanting to just pass out and get it over with. Sometimes the affect of chemo was everything combined while other times were fine. Well, maybe weak and shaky, but not violently ill. I never knew what to expect for sure.

The girls and I continued to live in Pocatello, Dick in St. Anthony, commuting back and forth as often as possible.

Our financial situation worsened each day as we fought to pay off the doctor and hospital bills and maintain living expenses. We lived, surviving from day to day. I would shake each time the phone rang. I knew it would be collection agencies, and I didn't have the money to give them nor the strength to deal with them. All too often, my daughters were left the awful responsibility of dealing with the collectors, a task they should never have had to do.

The girls worked as hard as they could to maintain the house, the yard, school, part-time jobs, and the activities in which they were involved. The house needed some touch up work done on it, and the yard needed weeding and mowing. Our lawn mower was broken and working in the sun would make the *chemo-sickies* even worse. I was sure the girls and I could maintain the house, but doing the heavy yard work seemed more than we could deal with.

My home teachers (elders in the church) visited and I asked them for help. They said they would see what they could do which was, evidently, to stop visiting. I never saw them again. I called the bishop and asked if he could have the scouts or elder's quorum help me with the yard. He said he would try, but I needed to remember that people were very busy. I never heard back from him.

Our lawn mower was broken so I borrowed one from my in-laws and Melissa got the lawn mowed while Leisl did laundry. Together the three of us picked up debris, leaves, and stuff out of the yard, loaded everything in the trunk of the car and hauled it to the garbage dump. My arm started to swell, felt tight and was painful. I called the doctor and he told me about lymphedema, which he said was natural after having a mastectomy that had disrupted the lymph system. He would phone in a prescription that should help. Great, more medication expense!

Within minutes of talking with the doctor, my in-laws phoned and told me they needed the lawn mower back right then so the twins could come down and get their lawn done. I asked if the twins could stop by my house and pick it up…after all, they had to drive past my house to get to theirs. No, I had borrowed it, so I needed to bring it back immediately. I told them Dick would be home in a few days and he could bring it down then and even mow the lawn for them. No, they had to have it right then. It was, after all, theirs and should have been returned sooner. Then they added, "we don't want you to forget where it belongs."

It made me so angry I slammed down the phone and began to cry. No one from the church would help. No one in the family would help us. It was hot and I was sticky and dirty from yard work. My arm hurt, and I was so emotionally frustrated I could scarcely stand it. I tore out of the house, opened the trunk, and had Melissa help me load the big heavy mower in the car. Together we drove over to their house, pulled the mower out of the trunk, and threw it out on the lawn. We got back in the car and I peeled away from their house, tires flinging dirt and gravel into the air, and maniacally yelled "shove it up your god damn butts" out the window, swearing to never return to their house. *Trust me,* I thought, *if I were going to steal anything at this time of my life, it would be money not a freakin' lawn mower.* I was sick of them all for telling everyone how pathetic we were, how sick I was, how much they did for me, and how badly they felt for us, when in actuality they chose to ignore us and say hurting things to us. I was tired of them feeling sorry for their son having to live and work hours away while we struggled to survive. I was sick of them telling my kids that we were not living the way we should be. And, I was damn sick and tired of a congregation that spoke of compassion, love and service rather than showing it.

As we approached the house, I finally gained a little control, stopped crying, blew my nose, wiped my eyes, and got brave enough to look at Melissa. She was sitting absolutely straight, forced against the seat, and appeared to be in shock. Needless to say, I felt stupid for having had such an emotional outburst over such a dumb thing.

"Well, I bet that was weird," was all I could say.

Melissa nodded, her eyes wide and complexion pale, and said, "Holy shit, Mom. Up their butts?"

We stared at each other, trying to establish a safe ground to be on. Did she really witness my out-of-control hissy-fit? Did she really say 'Holy shit' in front of me? Who or what had taken over our bodies and made them act so strangely? It was as if we were trapped in Twilight Zone and couldn't get out. Then, the absurdity of it all hit us. I tried to muffle a laugh that was creeping out of my mouth. It made more of a snort sound than a muffled laugh. Melissa giggled an absolutely nervous titter which made me laugh out loud. I laughed hard. Melissa roared with laughter. We laughed so hard we were crying. We rolled out of the car and hung on each other for support as we staggered our way into the house, tripped over ourselves and collapsed on the couch, gasping for air between loud guffaws of laughter.

"Hey, Leisl, ya' shoulda heard Mom tell Granny and Gramps to stick it up their butts. It was great!" Snort, laugh, wheeze!

"Shuddup, Melissa. It was awful. Just…(snort, wheeze, guffaw) awful!" We were totally out of control and it felt good!

Leisl just looked at us, shook her head in disbelief, and joined the insane laughter. She kept trying to ask what happened between gales of laughter, and we kept trying to tell her. The three of us laughed until we were weak.

Needless to say, I didn't hear from Dick's parents for nearly two weeks, and when they were finally ready to talk, we never mentioned the lawn mower incident.

One night I was alone in the house. Dick was in St. Anthony, the girls were at a dance, and the quietness became a dark threatening gloom. I felt as if the jaws of hell were opening for me. I stood in front of the mirror and robotically examined my body. There I was, bloated, pasty, and with broken and brittle hair that needed to be shaved bald. When I brushed it, it would fill the hair brush. I would awake in the morning with hair on my pillow. I would find it in the bathtub after I'd shower. I knew I should shave it off, but doing so would be the final admission that it really was cancer. I knew people died when they had cancer, and I wasn't going to give into it willingly. I came into the world a redhead, and if I had to leave the world, it would be with hair—and the hair would be red. Everyone told me that my hair would grow back in, thick, curly and beautiful, but I just couldn't do it. *Besides*, I reasoned, *I look awful in hats and scarves.* Thatches of hair were missing. The hair remaining did not look nor feel healthy, but it was mine.

My fingernails were broken, snaggy, and splitting down toward the quick. My skin tone was ghoulishly greenish-yellow. I removed my blouse and bra. I looked at my full frontal view, not to check the incision for healing, but to assess how Dick must see me. Part of me was gone. The purplish-red slash under my arm and across my chest where my breast used to be looked horrendously gross. The remaining breast only taunted the blob I had become.

I was filled with a dark anguished anger that is without description. I grabbed a bottle of hand lotion and flung it against the wall. I threw pillows, pictures, clothing, anything with in reach. I sobbed, my chest heaving with animal-like moans. Every cell in my body hurt. I shook until I couldn't stand.

I decided that Dick only touched me, or made love to me, out of pity. I couldn't live being pitied. I had ruined his life by making the selfish choice to live. If only I hadn't fought to live, Dick and the girls wouldn't be in this financial mess of unconquerable doctor, hospital, and living bills. They would have life insurance money to pay the bills and for the funeral expenses. They would have a chance to survive. I knew I would always be sick and they would soon become embarrassed and humiliated to be seen with me. I ran to the bathroom, vomiting. The vomiting soon turned to dry heaves and the crying subsided into sobbing.

A voice in the back of my mind taunted me—*"It doesn't have to be this way. You could end it now. You have enough pills to do it nicely. Just take them and crawl in bed. Everyone will think you just passed away in your sleep. It will be fine. Just do it. I'll stay here with you. C'mon, I'll be with you all the way.*

I found myself standing in the bathroom, holding a bottle of pills. Then another voice reminded me of a past conversation.

"It will be hard for you and everyone if you choose to stay. It will be easier if you come."

"I know, but I have to stay."

"Are you willing to stay knowing how hard it will be for you? For everyone?"

"Yes. I'm just not ready to go. I want to stay with Dick. I want to raise my daughters. I want to stay with them."

I put the lid back on the bottle and replaced it with the others in the medicine cabinet. I needed to hear Dick's voice. I called the facility in St. Anthony, hoping he would be at work rather than sitting in the motor home. They paged him over the radio, and in a few seconds I heard him say hello. I started to cry with relief.

"What's wrong, Sharon?"

"I needed to hear your voice. I can't make it without hearing you love me and need me and that you are glad I'm alive."

"I thank God everyday that you are alive, Sharon. I need you and I love you."

"I'm just so scared tonight. I need you so badly."

"I need you, too."

"I'll be fine now. I just needed to hear your voice. I miss you."

I hung the phone back in its cradle and finished undressing. I took a long hot bath, put on my nightgown, and crawled into bed, exhausted. I felt as if a loving Father in Heaven was scooping my emotional and spiritual body into His comforting arms, allowing it to gain renewed strength while my physical body curled up for a much needed, healing sleep. I felt protected and comforted with the knowledge that I was loved and that I would find the peace my inner self needed to be healed. I slept soundly and peacefully.

The girls woke me when they came home and asked if I was alright. I couldn't imagine why they were concerned until I looked around at the room I had devastated in my temper fit.

"Hmmmm, this looks pretty bad, doesn't it?"

"Yeh, Mom. What happened?"

"I had a bad night," I answered.

"Well," they responded. "you go make some cocoa and toast for us and we'll clean it up."

I knew they were remembering the lawn mower incident. They put the room back together, and we sat up long and late hearing about the dance, their friends, and making other mom-and-daughter talk. The devastated room joined the lawn mower in the land of things not discussed.

## Making Changes, Moving On

The house finally sold, but at a loss. We hadn't owned it long enough to have any equity in it. The previous owners had a second mortgage on it that was not discovered until we were attempting to get the paper work done to sell it. The mortgage company refused their responsibility for having sold it to us without resolving the second mortgage problem with the original owners, and we didn't have the money for a lawyer to fight it. We decided to cut our losses and just move. Meanwhile, the interest on the other expenses continued to grow.

Leisl was a senior and Melissa a junior in high school when we moved to St. Anthony. They had built wonderful lives in Pocatello and were angry and sad that we were leaving, but we were a family and we were going to stay a family if it killed us, and it nearly did.

We moved into a rental house out in the country that was at the end of a long unpaved driveway. It was October 15$^{th}$ and it started to snow as we unloaded the moving van. The snow compounded daily never taking time to melt away between storms. I couldn't remember ever seeing that much snow. A wonderful neighbor, Scotty, would plow the driveway for us everyday. Without his generosity, I would not have survived living there.

Once a week I would escape our winter prison and drive to Pocatello for chemo therapy. The reaction to the treatments became more severe. I would leave early the mornings of treatment day hoping that I could get back home before the reaction hit me. I was so sick one day that all I could do when I got home was to open the car door, fall out into the snow, kick the door shut, and crawl to the walkway and up the stairs. I pulled myself up to the doorknob, let myself in, and crawled to the bathroom where I was very, very ill. I was sick all week that time, and when I went down the following week for treatment, I was so anemic that the next round of chemo was postponed for two weeks. I knew chemo was the only way I was going to beat this evil cancer thing, so I was terrified to miss even one treatment. My entire focus was on testing and treatments to get well even if it was at the expense of my emotional, spiritual, and psychological health. I had to have those chemo treatments. I had to stay alive. I spent the next two weeks resting and eating all the good things we know we should.

I continued to study basic reading, word recognition, pronunciation, and reading comprehension. I read, and re-read, and then wrote what I read. I practiced writing words, then sentences. Frustration became a daily companion that taunted me with my inabilities.

Then one day, Melissa simplified the learning task for me when she said, "Geez, Mom. What's the big deal? You learned all that once before and you were just a little kid. Surely you can do it now you're an adult."

Her teenage wisdom changed my perspective of the learning process I was facing. By dang, if a little kid can learn it with no pre-knowledge of it, I really could do it. I knew how once and I could make the mind bring it back to me. We went to the library and checked out books. We read Dr. Seuss, poetry, easy books and soon novels. If someone would pronounce a word while I was looking at it, it would stay in memory. So, word by word, it all started coming back to me.

I would sit on the couch or out on the front porch and read to the dog, Aggie. The poor old thing would sit by me, tipping her head with her ears raised appropriately to the sound of my words, as I read aloud listening to the roll of the words.

Dick and I would go for long drives in the country and I would read to him, sounding out the words I no longer recognized. He would correct the pronunciation, and give a definition when needed.

Christmas was approaching and we had nothing to offer. I found a store that would let me come in after hours and vacuum and clean in exchange for clothing articles for the girls for Christmas. It was hard for me to do, but I could work at my own pace and take time, without audience, to meet the demands inflicted by the chemo therapy. I could sleep long during the day to recuperate and feel I was contributing to the family. The girls received jeans, tee shirts, sweaters, jewelry, and even new coats for Christmas that year.

We survived living at the end of a country lane that winter, being plowed out daily, while watching the snow mounds grow higher and deeper. Then, one day, the snow began to melt and I started planning how to move into town. I found a big six bedroom, four bathroom house and in April we moved. I knew there would still be snow next winter, but I knew the city would remove it as it fell. At least, I hoped they would.

Springtime brought warm sunshine, flowers and gentle breezes instead of freezing wet and bone-chilling winds. I actually started feeling stronger and more hopeful. I loved the days when Dick would take me fishing. I would sit in a lawn furniture lounge chair, wrapped in a blanket, and watch him wade the stream, casting his fly line with a poetry no words can express. The muscles in his shoulders and arm would ripple with each cast. He would turn now and then to check on how I was and to send a reassuring smile in my direction.

When he had caught three or four trout, he'd wade in, set up the little camp stove and cook them with potatoes and onions and we would feast on them as we watched the river, trees, and the circling osprey. The warmth of the sunshine, the fresh breezes, and the joy of togetherness added greatly to the healing process. John Denver was so right when he sang "Sunshine on my shoulders makes me happy…almost always make me high."

Our finances were still an unconquerable mess that resulted in us filing for bankruptcy. Demoralizing as it was, it was also a relief to be able to answer the phone without fear. We would pay back everything as we could, but at least it wouldn't be on our shoulders, bearing down on us every waking minute.

I decided I needed more help with learning, so I applied for the teacher's aide position at the Youth Services Center. Some how or other, I bluffed my way through the interview and was offered the job. I was both delighted and terrified. I talked with the Director of Education and arranged to come in early to review the material that would be assigned to the students. I would learn it, and then I would help students learn it. Learning and then teaching something is a sure way to retain it. It was a perfect arrangement.

I completed a year of weekly chemo therapy treatments. I used sick leave as quickly as it was earned, but I survived the treatments and worked hard when I could be there. I loved my job but soon found myself wanting new challenges, more difficult tasks, and a higher demand of my knowledge.

I applied for the Education Secretary position that came open and was offered the job. I had completed a two-year program business college, as well as numerous other college classes, and felt it was time to reclaim that part of my life. My first day on the job in the office was absolutely terrifying! There I sat facing a big black ominous Olivetti electric typewriter, and I had no clue what to do with it. I was sure I'd be fired before the day was over. I looked around the office and found an operator's manual for the Olivetti. Hmmm, I can do this.

I eventually got it turned on, sat in front of it, wiggled my fingers around, and found the first key to push. I started to press keys down to write a memo as requested by the director. Thank goodness he was really busy and didn't realize that it took me all morning to type three sentences.

I found a paper keyboard and instructions for what fingers to use for which keys, practiced the correct finger placement and movement, and memorized the keyboard. Within weeks, I reclaimed most of the skills I had learned in school and business college.

I loved the learning process and the controlled social atmosphere of work where I could meet people and make new friends. Wonderful people daily shared their fresh ideas, stories, experiences, and challenges with me. Before long, I gained confidence and the self-esteem that comes from feeling productive. I was growing stronger, learning new things, and discovered that others not only expected things from me, but knew they could count on me. These new workplace acquaintances didn't know who I had been, they didn't know what I had been through, and they didn't expect anything from me but the best. It was wonderful. How grateful I was to be recognized as a real live contributor.

# Invitation to Healing

Sara, one of my new friends, invited Dick and me to a Christmas party. We were still reeling from the bankruptcy. We had no money. We had no new nice clothes to wear, and our Christmas spirits were buried in the bah-humbugs of Christmas survival. We were struggling to keep a roof over our heads and food in the house. How could we enjoy Christmas when there was no money for daily needs, let alone for holiday decorations, baking goods, and gifts?

Living in a survival mode had blinded us to the wonderful gifts of the season. Our inner spirits were broken. We were becoming bitter, heavy-hearted, and cynical. We didn't like who we were becoming, but hadn't the inner strength to change. We had little to offer others, but we were severely in need of being cheered. We needed to find a way to change our attitudes from despair and worry before the stress of it all caused us more illness and pain. We needed to find a *normal*, more reality-based way to live. So, we accepted the invitation with a desperateness that overcame the fear of being with others in a party setting.

We dressed in the best we had, which was moderately okay, got in our rattle-trap car, and braved the cold winter night and icy roads. We soon found ourselves parked in front of Sara's home, wondering if we were ready for a cozy social gathering. I was so nervous I nearly threw up when Dick said, "Let's go in." It took all the courage I could muster to get out of the car and walk towards their front door.

Sara's face lit up when she opened the door to us. "I'm so glad you came! Come in and make yourself comfortable. Here, let me introduce you to everyone." The house was warm, beautifully decorated, and it felt good to be there. It was an evening that I'll never forget.

The party was a unique experience. Instead of the usual holiday conversation and gift exchange, we enjoyed several musical presentations and then we all joined our voices together and sang Christmas carols. The room was bright with the joy of the Season as we sang the songs:

*Silent night, holy night; all is calm, all is bright.*
*O Come all ye faithful, joyful and triumphant.*
*O Holy Night, the stars were brightly shining.*
*O Come, O Come Emanuel.*

And,

*Away in the manger, no room for a bed…*
*Be near me, Lord Jesus, I ask Thee to stay*
*Close by me forever, and love me, I pray;*
*Bless all the dear children in Thy tender care,*
*And take us to heaven to live with Thee there.*

Peaceful songs. Healing songs. Tears filled my eyes, and my voice choked. How can one sing those beautiful songs of peace and still feel anger toward others?

*God forgive me, and help me to learn to forgive others. Carrying hurt and anger is too heavy of a burden for anyone to be saddled with.*

For the first time in several years, I felt the companionship of the Comforter who once stood by my side in the CCU, and recognized that this Being was there to help me with the next step in my decision to live.

*Lead me. Guide me. Walk beside me…Help me find the way.*

I had chosen to stay alive. Now that I had survived, I had to decide how to live a quality life that was deserving of all I had been given. I found myself face to face with the fact that my anger towards those who had hurt, shunned or caused me emotional pain was not founded on the spiritual beliefs I professed to live. I said I believed in forgiveness, but I was carrying around so much anger-and-hurt-baggage that I had turned my back on many of my own personal beliefs. I came face-to-face with my own shortcomings, and I didn't like it at all. I resolved to let it go, and to move on.

Our hearts softened as we sang, and opened up to all the good things there are in life. The warmth of friendship and sharing, the aroma of fresh-baked delicacies mixed with the fragrance of oranges, tangerines, and pine that had intoxicatingly led us into the true spirit of the holidays. This wonderful new friend, Sara, had sensed our need and opened the door for spiritual healing. And, my Comforter-friend smiled, knowing I had made a good choice in deciding to remain with Dick and the girls. For the first time in quite a while, we felt peaceful and calm.

*Silent night. Holy night.*
*All is calm. All is bright.*

As we drove home after that most pleasant experience, we reveled in the inner peace we felt. We commented on how hardened we had allowed ourselves to become. We resolved to never allow ourselves to get into that miserable trap of negativity again. The gentleness we enjoyed at Sara's party reminded us of another Christmas that was made memorable by the true spirit of the holidays.

Dick had received military orders to LaMaddelena, Sardinia, Italy and had to leave a few months before the girls and I were able to make the move. He had to settle in, secure housing, and give our household goods time to be shipped there before we were allowed to join him.

I had purchased Christmas and Santa gifts for the girls and had mailed them to Dick early in November. The girls and I flew to Italy the last part of November where we lived in a hotel waiting for everything to arrive so we could move into a house. We checked the mail daily, watching for the wonderful Christmas presents to arrive.

On Christmas Eve day, one box of the many that were mailed arrived. Just one. It had two pair of scissors, a doll house but no dolls, a Barbie doll bicycle but no Barbie doll, a cardboard nativity scene with paper doll figures, and two pair of gloves. That was all. Living in the hotel was costly and we only had a small amount of money.

We left the girls with the family that owned the hotel and ran for town, arriving just as the stores were closing. We were able to buy some tangerines and oranges and two dolls—nothing more. Our hearts hurt for our little girls. We wondered how they would handle being away from grandparents, cousins, and friends only to have an all but empty Christmas in a foreign county. We trudged up the stairs in the hotel to our rooms and opened the door to the most beautiful sight in the world.

The family that owned the hotel helped the girls find a broken pine bough and helped them to hang it from the ceiling so it would look like it was standing up like a Christmas tree propped on a table. They had decorated this make-do Christmas tree with paper cut-outs and colored pictures, and had even made a lop-sided star for the top. Beneath the tree was the paper Nativity scene with poor bent Joseph and Mary, a wrinkled manger bed and babe, and an assortment of un-folded and hand-pressed animals…donkey, cows, camels and sheep. It was beautiful. Our eyes filled with tears of pride and thankfulness, and the smell of tangerines, oranges and pine wafted through our little suite of rooms as we sat on the floor listening to the girls reciting the story of Christmas. How wonderful to have children to remind us of what is important and needed! The unimportant things, the presents, arrived a few days later.

And here we were again, thankful to have had the true spirit of Christmas surround us when we needed it most. Attending Sara's wonderful party was yet another step in the healing process. It renewed our faith.

# The Wonderful World of Work

Work continued to be a healthy challenge. I read office books and manuals on filing systems, ergonomics, office procedures, and so forth, and implemented what I read. Lost knowledge was returning at a rapid pace and I was elated to be functioning and earning money. I resolved to become the best office professional possible. I determined to make work an on-going learning experience, not just mentally and as a partial solution to our financial problems, but also as a source for building friendships and increasing social activities.

The more skilled I became, the more I demanded of myself. I located a professional organization called Professional Secretaries International (PSI) that met monthly in Idaho Falls, which was an hour drive from St. Anthony. I felt and looked like frump-girl when compared with their poise. My hair was still dry and brittle, my skin still looked pukey-green, and I was still bloated from the prednisone that I was still taking. Still, still, *still*. But the word *still* was no longer a whine or an unending bad thing. It was a reminder that I was alive and had a lot of reasons to stay alive, to 'still' be alive.

I wasn't sure this group of professionals wanted me as a member, but I was going to be one. I paid my dues and dragged myself to the meetings, determined to learn all they knew.

A soon to become friend, Eileen, initiated and welcomed me into the Eagle Rock Chapter of PSI. I met new friends—Vicki and Chris, also members of this organization who encouraged me to volunteer for committees. I read the committee guidelines, learning how to do whatever the committee needed to accomplish. After two years of committee work, I decided to run for chapter treasurer. I hadn't balanced my own checkbook forever, mostly because money issues terrified me after what we had recently survived. I served as treasurer, the next year as president-elect, and the following year as president of the Eagle Rock Chapter of PSI.

During the year I was the chapter's president-elect, I decided to take the exam for Certified Professional Secretary, a certification offered through PSI. It involved taking a two-day exam at Idaho State University in Pocatello, Idaho that covered Economics, Accounting, Business Law, Office Technology, Office Administration, Business Communication, Behavioral Science in Business, Human Resource Management, and Organizations and Management. I studied long and hard for a full year, an hour each morning before getting ready for work, two hours each evening six days a week, taking only one day off from the studying regime. I spent the day off from my study routine telling Dick, the girls, sales clerks, cashiers, and any-and-every-one I met what I had learned to reinforce it in my own mind. I read manuals aloud in the car while Dick drove. I studied my notes in the lines at the store or post office. Then, the first of May, Vicki and I took the test and began the long six weeks wait for the results.

Dick phoned one day in mid-June to say he had picked up the mail and had the test results. He asked if I wanted him to bring them over to my office. I was so nervous I knew I couldn't, or wouldn't, open the envelope at work. I didn't want others there in case I had failed. It would be devastating to know that I hadn't been able to retain all the reading and studying long enough, or well enough, to pass the exam. I knew I would feel really stupid and inept, and would probably cry. I also knew I would do an uncontrollable happy dance if I passed and that could prove to be just as scary as failing and, once again, I would probably cry.

Yet, I couldn't stand to not know how I had done. I asked him to open it and read it to me. He read off the results of each of the six exams one by one with the scores. I placed in the upper range of 96th/98th percentile in all subjects but one. I was in the 78th percentile in Accounting, which wasn't great, but it was passing. I had passed the CPS exam on the first attempt. I was elated to say the least. I now knew for sure that I could learn anything, read and write anything I wanted, and had no need to be embarrassed or feel small again, ever.

# The Butties, and Other Growth Experiences

Soon after taking the exam, I met Julie and Kay (also members of the PSI) who, along with Vicki and Chris, became the Butties. We instantly became friends for life. We went to all the conferences together, played hard and laughed a lot. Once, when I was unable to get off work for a training conference, the four of them went without me. They sent me cards telling of all the fun things they were doing, and how much they missed me being there. One of the cards showed five people sitting at a lunch counter, trousers pulled low showing butt cracks. Each had written a message and their name on 'the butt of their choice', leaving one good-sized lily-white moon butt unclaimed. The five of us have been the 'Butties' ever since then.

With much encouragement from the Butties, I decided to continue being actively involved in PSI by running for a higher office. I went on to serve as treasurer, president-elect, and eventually president for the Utah-Idaho division of PSI. During my year as president, the division expanded to include Oregon.

It was during my affiliation with Professional Secretaries International (now known as International Association of Administrative Professionals) that I further developed confidence, increased self-esteem, and came to trust in others outside my immediate family once again. I developed not only professionally but also personally. I met extremely dedicated people who were/are committed to excellence. Their association not only helped me keep abreast of the trends and technology needed in the workplace, but also afforded avenue to make many wonderful, life-long friends.

When I was ill, I wanted to live. I wanted everyday I lived to be better than the previous day had been. As I sorted through my emotions, feelings, and experiences, I found remnants of who I had once been. And, I found a dream of who I wanted to become. I prayed to find growth experiences and people who could help me become a better person. Answers to prayers often come in strange ways.

Invitations to speak, lead workshops, and give presentations at seminars hosted by a variety of professional organizations, church groups, and other agencies started coming my way. The first invitation I received was frightening to accept. I knew words still slipped out of mind a millisecond after I opened my mouth to speak, but I had to see if I could stand up in front of a group and say something of any importance. I had to see if I had the guts to have a room full of people look directly at me for a given time without me getting self-conscious or flustered.

I had to know if I really believed in myself.

The beginning 30 minutes or so of that first workshop went just fine, and then it happened. Mid-sentence of a dramatically important impact statement, I lost the word I needed. Panic gripped for a brief moment. *What should I do? Should I just walk away, out of the building, change my name and move to outer Mongolia?* I decided in that millisecond-of-time that this was a do-or-die thing. Without the quick return of that stinkin' word, I had nothing to do but bluff my way through. I kicked into the drama-mode, acted like it was a pause for emotional reflection, and waited for the word.

It never came.

I forced myself to stay calm, and just in time, another suitable word popped in to my mind and came out my mouth. It worked, and I completed the workshop with renewed enthusiasm. People even applauded long and loud for me at the conclusion, and came up to tell my how much they had enjoyed it. Wow! I was living on a high cloud that day!

I am very proud of where I came from, who I was, what I have experienced, what is happening today, and who I have become. I no longer worry if my prosthesis looks normal, nor if my shirt hangs weird. I choose not to waste my time mountain-climbing over molehills. I rejoice in friendships, family, love and caring. I enjoy meeting people and making new friends. I value the positive contributions that others have made to make life more cherished.

St. Anthony is still my home. I still work in the education program at the Juvenile Corrections Center, formerly known as the Youth Services Center. The Juvenile Corrections Center works with Idaho's incarcerated, at-risk youth. The staff are dedicated professionals who do all they can to ensure that the youth placed at our facility make the changes necessary to become responsible members of the community to which they are returned. I am proud to be included as a member of that outstanding group of professionals.

# Happily Ever After...

Dick and I have been married nearly forty years. My girls are grown, leading lives of their own. I have three wonderful grandchildren—Rachel, Coda, and Tylar Kristina—all whom I adore. I have one dog and a cat. My life feels balanced and I am happy.

Dick still works at the Juvenile Corrections Center, too. He also writes a column for a wonderful weekly newspaper, The Island Park News (**www.islandparknews.com**. You'll find his column in the Crackerbarrell section as Marler's Musings or at **www.Sowerss.com**). You may even find samples of his photography, which is becoming well recognized. He is still tall, handsome, and charming, and I am as crazy about him as I was the day I married him. We have been best friends since we were kids.

Dick and the girls were also victims of cancer. Not of the disease itself, but of all the things associated with it. You see, there are always more victims of cancer than just the one who is ill. Mates worry as they try to be good support without denying the victim the opportunity to make the decisions or do the tasks they used to do, and are still capable of doing. They worry that they are expecting too much, not being as supportive as they need to be, and they feel guilty and angry. Guilty that they are well and you are not. Angry that you are sick and they can not make you well. Guilty if they worry about their own adjustments to life...*what will I do without him or her, how can I support the kids, will I be able to keep the house, the job, our way of life?* Angry that the fairy tale of happily ever after didn't come true.

Children, young or old, think about life without the mother or father, the sister or the brother, and they worry over what will happen to them. Many take on adult roles, trying to make it all better by assuming too many responsibilities for a child.

Our daughters have made adjustments to the scars they gathered during our family's cancer experience. They are strong, resilient, and beautiful young women who strongly believe in yearly checkups and health maintenance. Their lives have had ups-and-downs, just like your life and mine. They have well proven that they can handle the deep pits of hell as well as the golden beams in their own lives. They are remarkable women with survival stories of their own. Their stories could fill a book, but those stories are for them, not me, to tell.

I have been cancer-free for 20 years, and oddly enough, I find myself thinking of how blessed I have been to have had this learning experience, and to rediscover what I know to be true. The reaffirmation of fundamental beliefs is a rewarding growth opportunity. I discovered many things about myself. Most importantly, I discovered that I love deeply and that I am deeply loved.

My story isn't just a story about surviving cancer. I think of it more as a story of living life, of building strength, resiliency, determination, and love based on a strong desire to regain a healthy and whole life. Strength and resiliency come from daring to try again when you have failed or experienced a set-back…and if needed, try and try again. Determination comes when you can no longer tolerate wallowing in self pity and absolutely know there is something better for you if you want it badly enough. And love is earned by learning to understand and forgive others and self.

As I went through the healing process, I found myself face to face with an issue I didn't want to give audience. I realized that my anger towards those who had hurt, shunned, or caused me emotional pain was not founded on what I professed to believe. I had always said that I believed in forgiveness, but I was carrying around so much *anger-and-hurt-baggage* that I had turned my back on a lot of my own personal beliefs. It was difficult for me (1) to admit that I was not living what I said I believed, and (2) to realize that I was just as wrong, if not more so, for holding to any real or perceived injustice. I had to choose to let it go and to move on. I re-discovered what I had already known…there is more to getting well than physical healing.

I have finally been able to internalize the concept that we all make mistakes and that we all have judged another unfairly. I have learned to forgive myself and others and have realized the importance of peacemakers in the world. I have also realized and internalized the concept that there is a time to stand firm in what you know to be right. I love the movie about the make-believe world of Camelot, particularly when King Arthur is explaining the need for a round table where knights could meet and talk. He stresses that 'might does not make right; right makes might'. All we need to do to have peace and harmony is to do what is right. We know that, don't we? Why would we want to live any other way? Why can't life be that simple? And why can't our world leaders create such a place to live?

I hope you are reading this because you need the motivation to get a mammogram. However, IF you are reading this because you currently are battling cancer, I pray you will find the strength to fight and overcome.

If you are not able to win the fight against cancer, leave a legacy of love with those you leave behind. Help them cope with losing you. Talk with them. Let them know they will not be alone. Let them help you face leaving this world for another with dignity and grace. Leave a legacy of peace, love, and of making the world a better place because you were a part of it. Help them accept what is happening to you and to them. Enlist them in accepting and in resolving to carry on your love of life in what they do in their lives.

We all come to an 'accepting' part of life when we examine who we are and how we think. I am not aware of the exact minute that I started to accept that person in the mirror years ago on that dark night of genuine despair. You know the one I'm talking about—she had crappy hair, skin, shape, and out-of-balance chest. She was sick, and sad, and so afraid of *life-as-it-was* that she considered removing herself from the lives of those she loved the most. She was my negative side, who thrived on the fatigue, worry, and illness.

Some how or other along the way, this negative force found a way to reach out to the real me from within the inner mirror of darkness in which we sometimes place ourselves. I took a chance and reached in to take her hand and pulled us into one being who was determined to heal the total person. We faced other dark episodes of warring over who would climb victoriously on the battle mount to declare a win, but no war as frightening as that brief period of time when death seemed a better bargain than life. We, the negative and positive factions of my being, faced many other challenges and enjoyed tremendous moments of success. Sometimes the dark side of her doom and gloom would pull me down. Other times, I would pull her up to a winning position. I'm not the only one that had faith in her ability to reclaim a good life. My husband and daughters set the winning course. Some friends and family may have abandoned me, but I made new friends who were willing to reach through the fear of rejection, and offer their protective encouragement which led me to a renewed belief in self. I was returning to a life of healthy, peaceful Oneness of spirit, hope, and happiness.

I appreciate the many strong people I have met over the past years who have lent me their strength when I needed it by telling their own stories of survival. I invite you to visit the MammySlammy site on the Internet at **www.mammyslammy.com** to not only read how others' have celebrated at their parties, but also to read some amazing stories of courage that people have shared with me. Let me share a few of their comments with you.

Mara who had breast cancer wrote of her experience: "Cancer was a dramatic experience for me. It was not easy, but it was worth living it and I would not change it if I had the opportunity to do so."

Bobbe, (a divorced mother with four sons), who had kidney cancer wrote: "Cancer is always in the back of my mind now along with the fact that I have only one kidney to function with. These two factors change one's lifestyle significantly. I am more conscious about what goes in my mouth, and about what comes out of my mouth (how I speak to and about others) since this experience. I have been cancer free for 16 months and I have three years and nine months to go before they boost my survival rate even higher."

Nate, Bobbe's teenage son, wrote: "My mom's road to recuperation was slow but progressive. But she was getting a little better everyday. Soon she was going to work again and back on her 'schedule'. All and all, my mom is a pretty tough woman. She likes to be called a survivor."

Katie, the teen who sang at the Relay for Life, had her story told by her sister. Carrie wrote: "Katie needs five years of clean MRI's to be considered in remission. But with the help of her family and friends, it will happen. Making new friends along the way, Katie took it all in stride. Never once during her long and arduous treatment, did Katie lose hope. With each new thing that was presented, she met it head on and never gave up hope. Her story is truly inspiring."

Steve, a survivor of lung cancer wrote of his experience: "So much happened in 2002. I have so much to be grateful for. Being innocently loved by a very young granddaughter. Having a son wake us up so we could be in charge of our own destiny. Being prayed for by so many.

Knowing that doctors aren't always right but, dang we're glad to have them. Being able to keep an attitude that we could beat this thing. Being able to stay physically strong enough to overcome some serious insults to my body. Learning that doing the weekly vacuuming is only a start and that staying healthy means giving and supporting your caregiver. Being able to say cancer without a bad reaction. Proving that you knew you'd pull through all along. Knowing that you are so very, very lucky. Knowing that you have the best wife anyone could possibly have. Gee, 2002 was a very good year!"

Sara's story is one praising the early detection of breast cancer through mammography. She insists her breast cancer was "no big deal" but it truly is. She hadn't been in for a yearly checkup for sometime and had never had a mammogram. She promised her daughter that she would make an appointment and she did. Her cancer was detected while in the early stages and was taken care of with a lumpectomy and radiation. Sara wrote in her story: "This brush with cancer literally became the beginning of new life for me. I have chosen to live more expressively, more fully, more gratefully…and more carefully (regular checkups and mammograms). I take nothing for granted."

And my daughters?

Leisl wrote a piece on June 25, 2001, for an editorial column titled, Just Something To Think About. "One more month lump free. This is once again the result of my monthly ritualistic self breast exam. I am a big believer in these and I never miss a month. After all, if it weren't for early detection, my mom would have died of breast cancer. Luckily, she caught it early. And she survived.

I know many people are embarrassed by just the thought of touching or even looking at themselves there. Get over it! There are so many cancer deaths that can be prevented by early detection and treatment. Right now, according the American Cancer Society, 'The 5-year relative survival rate for people with cancers for which the ACS has specific early detection recommendations (breast, colon, rectum, cervix, prostate, testis, oral cavity, and skin) is about 81%.' However, 'if all Americans had early detection testing according to ACS recommendations, the 5-year relative survival rate for people with these cancers would increase to about 95%.' That's an increase of 14%! Wow!

Not all cancers can be detected by self exams, true, but so many can. Get to know your body—what looks right, what feels right. Be aware of bumps and lumps and discolorations. Get yourself checked by your doctor every year. Stay current on your tests (Pap, thyroid, colonoscopy, mammogram). Your children will thank you."

Melissa put the icing on the cake with the following: "In my 20's I found a lump in my breast. Talk about scared!!! It did end up being nothing. Thank goodness. Since my 20's I have done monthly breast exams. I know *the girls* more than I care to admit. I willingly signed up for a mammogram at age 30 and will go back at 35. I still believe that my childhood, adolescence and life were normal. Bad things just happen sometimes. They are horrible, and you wonder if you will get through them. Then you turn it over to God. You can worry about it, you can take precautions, you can eat right, exercise, and do everything you can to ensure well being but when it comes right down to it, you have to leave the ultimate decisions to God and deal with life as it unfolds to you. If you treat your life as normal, it becomes so for you. It may not be easy or wonderful but it will be normal and you will be able to deal with it. Things can always get worse, but you can always adapt, deal with it, and get on to better days. Overall, life is what you choose to make it. Determine to live it to the fullest and to thank God for each and every day you have to live."

(Sigh, aren't they both wonderful?)

They all have success stories of their own. Drop in to **www. mammyslammy.com** and read about them. They are people who are strong and courageous. They are gentle people who care deeply for their family and friends. They are intelligent people, who take care of themselves. They are people like you and I, who love life and choose to live it to the fullest.

I have also met women who have made fear-based comments, such as: "I found a lump in my breast that I need to have checked out someday. I'm just too busy right now, but I will make an appointment as soon as my life settles down." Another said to me, "I have to admit that I have thought about getting regular mammograms, but it takes so long. I don't have time." Or, "I'd make an appointment for a mammogram, but I'm afraid they might find something." I'm sure you already know my answers to them.

"Foolish!"

"Silly!"

"Absurd!"

And, "You've got to be kidding."

Then I realized that they were using time and foolishness as a protective shield. They were not just procrastinating, they were genuinely afraid of the 'what might be'. It was the same fear that drove me to plan and hold the first MammySlammy.

Many talk shows have been, and will be, dedicated to the importance of mammograms. We know the American Cancer Society recommends mammogram screening every year for all women age forty-and-older. For those with risk factors, including a close family member who had breast cancer, annual mammograms should begin 10 years earlier than the age at which the relative was diagnosed. I was diagnosed at the age of forty; therefore, my daughters should get a yearly mammogram from age thirty on.

(*Leisl and Melissa, you have done so well with this, and I am so proud of you. Keep listening to your mother!*)

## Awareness to Action

We have all become quite well versed in the reasons for mammograms. Our only problem seems to be actually making and keeping an appointment. Why make it a chore, or a most unpleasant "have to do"? Why not make it a party?

Let me share a note from a participant in the MammySlammy events. Dixie, who participates yearly, wrote the following: "I am so grateful for the opportunities I have had to participate in the MammySlammy parties. I challenge others to find ways to make mammograms not only a yearly event, but a celebrated yearly event. The older I become, the more I celebrate life, not just my life, but that of those who have overcome and/or endured the trials they have been given. I feast on their strength, love their zest for life, and admire their attitudes as they choose to face the challenges and opportunities life offers. God bless us all!"

So, how do you get started with your plans? Just decide to do it. Resolve to take a leadership role in ensuring your own health, and the health of your friends. Pick up the phone, call your best friends and tell them what you have in mind. Ask them to come with you. Ask them to invite others to join you. Make a list of everyone who is invited. Check with your area imaging center or hospital, wherever you go for mammograms, and set up a party. It's that easy.

Remember that each woman will need to have her doctor fax or phone in a prescription to the X-ray center requesting the mammogram. Each participant will be required to call in, identify herself as a member of the MammySlammy Party, and provide contact information, the name of her doctor, and her insurance provider, or means of payment. Once that is done, plan the details your day. Be inventive and creative. Make it a memorable event in which others are excited to be included.

I am really excited to be thinking ahead to the next party, and the next, and the next. I can't help but wonder if others will start holding parties. What kind of activities will they do? Will someone have her life spared because of early detection? Will someone have the MammySlammy support system in place if they are detected with breast cancer? Is there more we could be doing to increase chances for survival?

During the interview conducted by Channel 8 News, I was asked what someone could do if they felt alone with no friends but wanted to participate in a MammySlammy. I suggested they attend ours. We were a group of friends and we had plenty of room for more. I invite you to adopt the same attitude and standard. It's true that it is fun to be with your established group of friends; but, it is even more enjoyable when each of those friends invites another friend you do not know so you can get acquainted with them. Making new friends enriches your life and gives you a stronger network should you need help in other areas. Reach out. Dare.

One of the definitions given in the Merriam-Webster's Collegiate Dictionary, Tenth Edition, for sisterhood is: "the solidarity of women based on shared conditions, experiences, or concerns." And so we now have the Sisterhood of the MammySlammy. Sign up today by enrolling others in the sisterhood by planning and holding a MammySlammy.

What are we going to do at our next party? Darned if I know yet! Tee shirts with catchy phrases like 'big boys don't get slammed' or 'I got slammed' or just a button with the word "Slammy" printed on it along with the year?

Maybe we'll design our own game. Queen Mammy instead of Old Maid? Slamo instead of Bunco? Slamo instead of Bingo? Maybe we'll make up our own board game.

Wow, the ideas just stack up unbelievably fast, don't they? We haven't decided or planned it out in detail, but I can promise you it will be the party of the year! What about yours?

We all know that a determined person can make a number of positive changes, but a combined force of determined people can change the world. Together we can make a difference.

Let's do it!

# Now...
# Write
# Your
# Story

*If I could tell you just one story*
*To make you smile today*
*It would be one of friendships shared*
*In, oh, so many ways*
*It would be a long, long story*
*That would warm a million hearts*
*But I don't have the words or rhyme*
*So you must write your part*

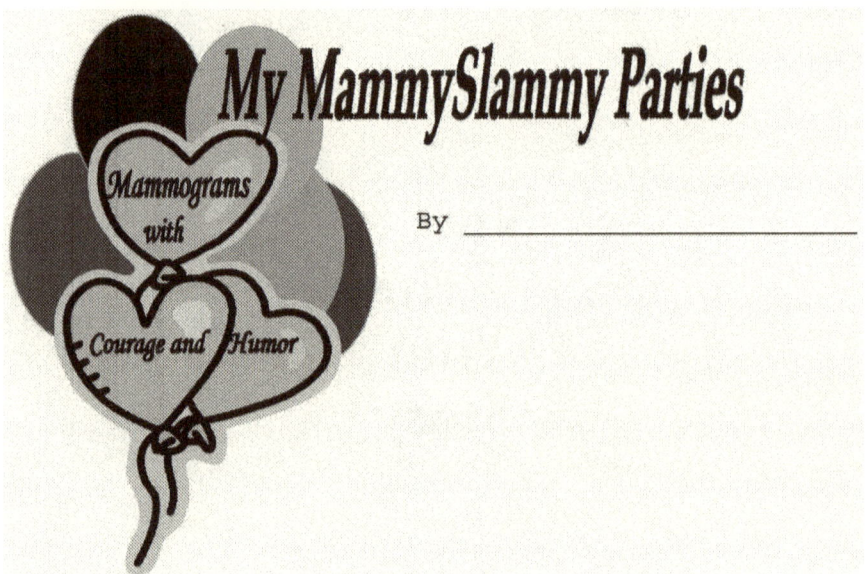

Use the next few pages to keep your personal journal. Use them to keep a list of those who participated so you can compare from one year to another. Record your activities...what did you do, what worked, and what didn't.

Use the successes to build on, and the less than successful activities to learn from.

Most of all, keep a journal of your feelings, your thoughts, and of any new ideas you gather from your MammySlammy. You are making your own history.

Be sure to check on our website for updates on what is happening there. Look for the great stories that are being shared, and lots of other wonderful ideas.

**MammySlammy Journal**                                      **Year 1**

Party Date: _____       Time: _____

Location: _____

Participants

| Name | Address | Phone | Email |
|------|---------|-------|-------|
|      |         |       |       |
|      |         |       |       |
|      |         |       |       |
|      |         |       |       |
|      |         |       |       |
|      |         |       |       |
|      |         |       |       |
|      |         |       |       |
|      |         |       |       |
|      |         |       |       |
|      |         |       |       |
|      |         |       |       |
|      |         |       |       |
|      |         |       |       |
|      |         |       |       |
|      |         |       |       |

**MammySlammy Journal**                                    **Year 1**

Activities, gifts, thoughts, ideas for next year, etc.

_____

_____

_____

_____

_____

_____

_____

_____

_____

_____

_____

_____

_____

_____

_____

_____

_____

_____

_____

_____

_____

**Journal Page 2**                                    **Year 1**

**Group Photographs**  **Year 1**

**Group Photographs**                                    **Year 1**

**MammySlammy Journal**                                      **Year 2**

Party Date: _____          Time: _____

Location: _____

Participants

| Name | Address | Phone | Email |
|---|---|---|---|
|  |  |  |  |
|  |  |  |  |
|  |  |  |  |
|  |  |  |  |
|  |  |  |  |
|  |  |  |  |
|  |  |  |  |
|  |  |  |  |
|  |  |  |  |
|  |  |  |  |
|  |  |  |  |
|  |  |  |  |
|  |  |  |  |
|  |  |  |  |
|  |  |  |  |
|  |  |  |  |
|  |  |  |  |
|  |  |  |  |

**MammySlammy Journal** Year 2

Activities, gifts, thoughts, ideas for next year, etc.

_____

_____

_____

_____

_____

_____

_____

_____

_____

_____

_____

_____

_____

_____

_____

_____

_____

_____

_____

_____

_____

_____

_____

_____

**Journal Page 2**                                    **Year 2**

_____

_____

_____

_____

_____

_____

_____

_____

_____

_____

_____

_____

_____

_____

_____

_____

_____

_____

_____

_____

_____

_____

**Group Photographs**  **Year 2**

**Group Photographs**                              **Year 2**

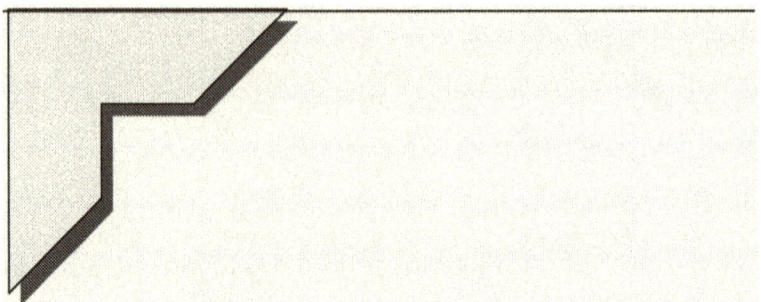

**MammySlammy Journal**                                      **Year 3**

Party Date: _____          Time: _____

Location: _____

Participants

| Name | Address | Phone | Email |
|------|---------|-------|-------|
|      |         |       |       |
|      |         |       |       |
|      |         |       |       |
|      |         |       |       |
|      |         |       |       |
|      |         |       |       |
|      |         |       |       |
|      |         |       |       |
|      |         |       |       |
|      |         |       |       |
|      |         |       |       |
|      |         |       |       |
|      |         |       |       |
|      |         |       |       |
|      |         |       |       |
|      |         |       |       |

**MammySlammy Journal**                                    **Year 3**

Activities, gifts, thoughts, ideas for next year, etc.

_____

_____

_____

_____

_____

_____

_____

_____

_____

_____

_____

_____

_____

_____

_____

_____

_____

_____

_____

_____

_____

**Journal Page 2**                                          **Year 3**

**Group Photographs**                                                    **Year 3**

**Group Photographs**                                              **Year 3**

# *Resources for additional information on breast cancer.*

There are many resources available today to help inform, enlighten and inspire those who seek them out. Knowledge is the hand that turns the doorknob so the guest can enter the room of healing.

Being aware of disease symptoms, methods of treatment, and expectations for survival, will help you become informed and involved in the maintenance of your own health. Resources can provide information. Doctors and hospitals can provide treatment. But it is up to you, to provide the courage and the determination to win your battle.

## Books:

Dr. Susan Love's Breast Book
by Susan M. Love, Karen Lindsey (Contributor), Marcia Williams (Illustrator), Susan M., Md. Love

Your Breast Cancer Treatment Handbook: Your Guide to Understanding the Disease, Treatments, Emotions and Recovery from Breast Cancer by Judy C. Kneece, Tricia Brown (Editor) (Paperback)

Living Beyond Breast Cancer: A Survivor's Guide for When Treatment Ends and the Rest of Your Life Begins by Marisa C. Weiss, Ellen Weiss (Paperback)

Be a Survivor: Your Guide to Breast Cancer Treatment (2nd Edition) by Vladimir Lange (Paperback)

Hope Is Contagious: The Breast Cancer Treatment Survival Handbook by Margit Esser Porter (Editor), et al (Paperback)

Helping Your Mate Face Breast Cancer: Tips for Becoming an Effective Support Partner for the One You Love During the Breast Cancer Experience by Judy C. Kneece (Paperback)

# Websites to visit:

www.cancer.gov            www.cancer.org

www.webmd.com            www.mammyslammy.com

0-595-27074-3